Dynamic Yoga

dynamic yoga

THE ULTIMATE WORKOUT THAT CHILLS
YOUR MIND AS IT CHARGES YOUR BODY

Godfrey Devereux

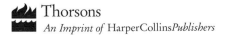

Thorsons
An Imprint of HarperCollins*Publishers*

Thorsons
An Imprint of HarperCollins*Publishers*
77–85 Fulham Palace Road,
Hammersmith, London W6 8JB

Published by Thorsons 1998

5 7 9 10 8 6 4

A catalogue record for this book
is available from the British Library

ISBN 0 7225 3657 7

Printed and bound in Great Britain by
Woolnough Bookbinding Ltd, Irthlingborough, Northants

This book is dedicated to the memory of Tirumalai Krishnamacharya for rescuing the ancient manual of classical hatha yoga, the Yoga Korunta, from oblivion and making it available to the modern world.

He did this both directly – in the form of Ashtanga Vinyasa Yoga through the work of his students K. Pattabhi Jois and B. N. S. Iyengar, both of Mysore – and indirectly in the form of Iyengar Yoga through the work of B. K. S. Iyengar of Pune, and in the form of Vinniyoga through the work of T. K. Desikachar of Madras.

Author's Note

Classical Hatha Yoga is by nature dynamic. Externally this is in the form of a flowing continuum between individual postures, and between postures, breathing and meditation. Internally it is in the profound, precise and continual activity of the body within the stillness of the postures. It is these dynamic qualities which make Hatha yoga meditation in action. Dynamic Yoga, then, is not another form of Hatha Yoga. It captures the essence of Hatha Yoga, as meditation in action, through emphasizing equally the internal and external dynamic of Hatha Yoga.

Contents

Acknowledgements

I would like to acknowledge the following teachers whose guidance has made Dynamic Yoga possible:

B. K. S. Iyengar of Pune and his students, for guiding me in the profound art of alignment

B. N. S. Iyengar of Mysore for guiding me in the traditional vinyasa krama of the Yoga Korunta

Swami Satyananda Saraswati and his students, for guiding me in the subtle art of the bandhas

I would also like to acknowledge the vital contribution of all of my students who have, even if unknowingly, contributed to the development of Dynamic Yoga

in particular Simon Turner and June Whittaker

I would also like to thank Sarah Robbie for her photographs and Simon Turner and Simon Lloyd for their willing and able assistance, Kirsten Heckterman for textual feedback

and finally Sarah Robbie and Louise White for their faith, support and friendship.

Caution

Dynamic Yoga, like all forms of Hatha Yoga, involves using your muscles, tendons, ligaments, joints and mind in novel and unfamiliar ways. While all of the movements are possible, and none of them is inherently harmful, you must be careful. Many of the movements are so different from those you are used to that you must approach them patiently and gradually. Do not rush, do not push, do not force your body. While you may get away with it sometimes, and with some parts of the body, at other times, and other body parts, you may not. Muscles once strained will soon repair: tendons and ligaments may not. Knees and necks are especially vulnerable.

Hatha Yoga is not simply a form of exercise. It is an extremely potent agent of transformation. The postures, the *bandhas* and the breathing, even when done partially or with difficulty, bring about deep changes in your energetic equilibrium. This can precipitate the release of deep psychic blocks. If these are not consciously met and allowed to resolve themselves they can have a disturbing effect on both mind and body. Take care to pay attention to what you are doing at all times, feeling its effect, and responding to that effect.

If you are suffering from any injury or illness, please consult both a medical professional and an experienced, trained yoga teacher before using this book. The therapeutic aspect of Hatha Yoga is one that should not be taken for granted. In order to use it for specific therapeutic purposes, a teacher fully trained and experienced in that application must be found. Such teachers are both rare and hard to find.

Preface

This book is a practical one. It describes an adaptation of the traditional method of Hatha Yoga. An adaptation developed and refined in hundreds of classes, with thousands of students, over many years. It presents a safe and effective integration of the techniques of Hatha Yoga, too often diminished by being separated. It has taken the form that it has on the basis of one criterion only: that it works. Whether or not it conformed to current practice, theory or dogma was not a concern. Whether people, of all ages and potential, could do it and benefit from it, was. Those of you who already practise will no doubt find in it points of familiarity. You may also find things unfamiliar, that might appear strange or irrelevant. However, if you try them you will find out, as many have before, that they all have their place.

For Hatha Yoga to work, it must respect the laws of body, movement, mind and consciousness that define the human being. So too Dynamic Yoga. But it does not present itself within the context of any belief system, dogma or religious perspective. In fact Hatha Yoga, like all forms of Yoga, does not require any beliefs, nor the expectations and limitations that they impose. Yoga is not a religion. You are not required to believe in any God or Gods, nor in reincarnation or karma. Yoga is a process that precludes the need for religion. It is a way of being: a means to clarify and reveal the nature of reality, and human existence. Once this is underway the need for religious guidance is unnecessary. All one needs is the practical advice of someone who knows the way. This book can provide you with some of that advice.

The specific methodology of Dynamic Yoga has developed through a process of interaction between my teachers and my students. With myself as its medium. It was the feedback from students, who did not necessarily have the same motivations or capacity as myself or my teachers, that brought

about the modifications to the traditional format that Dynamic Yoga represents. Many of my students made it clear that without such modification the practice and benefits of Hatha Yoga would be beyond them. It seemed to me churlish and unreasonable to adhere strictly to tradition if this puts yoga beyond the reach of all but the physically fit and deeply motivated. Yoga can benefit everyone, in more or less profound ways. This book makes it possible for those whose time, opportunity, motivation or capacity is restricted to enjoy some, at least, of the benefits of Hatha Yoga.

This book is offered to the reader in the hope that it might help to clarify the confusion that exists with regard to the different 'styles' of Hatha Yoga. It shows how each of the different emphases of the different styles fits into the single whole that is Hatha Yoga. It is not intended to be a different style, set aside from the others.

Ibiza, 1998

How to Use this Book

This book is divided into four parts. Part I gives you the theoretical background to understand what you will be doing.

Part II gives a detailed explanation of the technical processes involved in the practice.

Part III gives you details of the postures.

Part IV gives you the form of the practice.

In the Vinyasa section of Part III (page 68) you will find details of the moving part of the practice: Sun Salutations, Vinyasas and Vinyasanas. These are practised as part of both the Foundation and Preparatory Series. Before starting the Foundation Series, familiarize yourself with the Vinyasanas, Sukhasuryanamaskar and Sukhavinyasa. Before starting the Preparatory Series, familiarize yourself with Suryanamaskar and the Vinyasa.

In the Postures section (Part III), each posture is located over two opposite pages. On the left a large photograph shows the completed posture. Above is an explanation of key aspects of the pose. Below is a Summary description of the shape of the posture. On the right-hand page is a step by step verbal description of how to enter, establish, energize, hold and leave each posture. This text is supported by small photographs showing the various steps in and out of the posture and some details. When using this to learn a pose, read through to the end before trying the posture, referring back to it whenever you need to. You will also benefit from reading through these instructions at other times when not actually trying the postures.

In the Series sections of Part IV you will find graphic representations of the three Dynamic Yoga Series, and six short practice sequences. Whatever your experience, begin with the Pacifying Series, and progress though the Foundation Series to the Preparatory Series. The numbers accompanying each image refer to the posture and illustration number for that posture. The number will help you to find the detailed instructions and illustrations for each posture in Part III. These instructions must be complemented by a thorough grasp of the information in the technical section, Part II.

Read Part I first, then read Part II thoroughly, more than once. Do not be surprised or concerned if you find your reading of Part II overwhelming. It probably will be to begin with. But once you start to practise it will begin to make more and more sense. Once you have started to practise make sure you refer constantly to Part II, until you have fully embodied not only the specific information it contains, but also the principles underlying that information. Once you have done that you will be able to enjoy rapid, creative, autonomous practice safely and effectively.

When practising one of the Series you will need to find your way from posture to posture in the Postures section (Part III). With the exception of the Suryanamaskar postures the instructions for each pose show the next posture in the sequence for each Series. Each Series has its own symbol – ✦ for the Pacifying Series, ◼ for the Foundation Series, and ⬤ for the Preparatory Series – within which is a number referring to the next posture in that particular Series. Where a pose is used in more than one Series, take care to follow the correct symbol, double-checking with the Series layout (this does not apply to the six shorter sequences).

There are four stages to using this book to guide you in your practice:

1 Using the Series layout to find the postures in sequence, and then using the right-hand pages (which depict each movement in step-by-step photographs) as a guide.

2 Once you are familiar with the principles of entering, establishing, energizing, holding and releasing the postures, you can use the Series layout and the left-hand page of textual description to guide you.

3 Using just the Series layout and the main image.

4 Using just the Series layout.

Introduction

Yoga has lasted thousands of years because it works. Of all the approaches to yoga, Hatha Yoga is the most well known in the West. This is because of its comparative accessibility. Hatha Yoga works through the body. It involves moving the body into different and novel positions and relationships. These changes in the use of the body bring about changes in the mind. Rather than trying to effect the mind directly, which is far more difficult, Hatha Yoga allows us to work from the tangible, familiar arena of the physical body.

Hatha Yoga is the only approach to yoga that offers a wide range of physical benefits. While these are not the purpose of Hatha Yoga, they are unavoidable. In using the body to transform the mind, the body is also transformed. It is recalibrated, revitalized, harmonized: brought to a functional peak, both anatomically and physiologically, unreachable by any amount of diligent cross-training. It is these physical benefits that make it so popular. But, because these incidental physical benefits are connected to the intended psychological benefits, Hatha Yoga has a remarkable capacity to deliver far more than one might originally intend. Looking for a lithe, slim body, we also find a calm, clear mind. Hoping for strength and stamina, we also find increased determination and concentration. Wanting to be free of back pain, we find also freedom from compulsive anxiety. Seeking relief from asthma, we find also unlimited reserves of physical and mental energy. Trying to release tight shoulders and a stiff neck, we find also a new fund of enthusiasm and joy.

In fact Hatha Yoga is capable of delivering a remarkable range of benefits. These physical and mental benefits are not Hatha Yoga's primary purpose. This is simply to allow us to become fully in touch with who and what we are. This means not only our transient, conditioned characteristics, with which we only too easily identify. It also means our deeper, unconditioned nature, which we rarely even glimpse. It does this by bringing about a resolution of the conflict arising from the polarization of opposites within us. It allows us to experience, on every level of our being, the unity behind opposites, the relativity of all tendencies. Then we can see that by imposing a dualistic, either/or projection on reality we feel isolated, exposed and unsafe. The vulnerability of this dualistic projection generates the development of a complex and deeply embedded structure of tension, both mental and physical. This structure is designed to protect our vulnerability: to reduce the anxiety of being alive.

However this structure itself easily becomes the major hindrance to our living a full, joyful life. It does so by restricting movement: of body and of mind. Our ability to engage directly, fully and freely with the dynamic of life is hindered by deep layers of tension. Rigidity and inflexibility in body and mind restrict us to a limited range of responses to life. Hatha Yoga is designed to free us from all limitations. To do this it must dismantle these restricting structures through a simple, systematic recalibration of both body and mind. It does this through the agency of *asana* (alignment), *vinyasa* (connectivity), *bandha* (energetics), *pranayama* (breathing), and *drushti* (attentiveness). They are used to break down the patterns of holding and limitation from which we live. As this structure is dismantled, the deeper, profoundly rewarding aspects of our being are revealed.

The main Hatha Yoga techniques individually express one of the five fundamental energies of life. These energies are symbolized as space, air, fire, water and earth. Together they create an energetic model of the full potential of life. To use Hatha Yoga effectively, all these energies, and their techniques, must be used and balanced. Therefore

XIII

Dynamic Yoga not only presents each of these techniques carefully, precisely and practicably, but within the dynamic framework of their natural inter-relationship.

Hatha Yoga is a remarkably fruitful process. It can be given many different emphases, each offering quite different effects. It can be used as a form of exercise for developing a high degree of fitness. It can be used as a system of preventative, and even therapeutic medicine. It can be used as a form of relaxation. It can be used to develop a wide range of mental abilities. The various 'styles' of Hatha Yoga focus on a specific aspect and its effects: such as stretching for flexibility, continuity for stamina, or alignment for restructuring. This means that they offer only some of the benefits of yoga. Dynamic Yoga embraces and unifies the different styles and emphases into a single whole. Within this unity, the different parts are fulfilled in each other, without which even they, themselves, are likely to remain incomplete.

When Hatha Yoga is used, as intended, as a spiritual practice it encompasses and transcends all of its partial possibilities. Dynamic Yoga is a presentation of Hatha Yoga as a spiritual practice. It has as its practical aim a deep self-acceptance. This is based on self-knowledge, self-validation and self-empowerment. This means that it acts as a mirror to reveal to us exactly what we are, on every level of our being: physical, emotional, psychological, social, cultural, spiritual. We can then use this revelation to harmonize these different aspects of ourselves, and live our lives from the rich, integrated wholeness of our being.

Dynamic Yoga is a practical method. This book is designed to give you a series of progressive self-practice formats. These are based on the Classical Hatha Yoga Chikitsa. These are a group of basic yoga postures sequenced so as reharmonize the anatomical body. The Yoga Chikitsa postures were first popularized in the West by B. K. S. Iyengar, who reintroduced them as the foundation of safe,

effective Hatha Yoga practice. The Yoga Chikitsa format is known in the West as The Primary series of Ashtanga Vinyasa Yoga. This book contains three of the four Dynamic Yoga series that prepare for the safe, effective practice of that Series. They will allow you to progress gently and safely towards the more challenging traditional practice formats of Ashtanga Vinyasa Yoga, and other more advanced practices.

However, personal instruction in the subtleties of the techniques is indispensable. You will benefit, therefore, from finding teachers who can instruct you personally on the details of the practice, such as alignment, the *bandhas*, entering and leaving the postures, and breathing. This should not, however, become a substitute for self-practice. It is only within the silent experience of your own physical and mental structures that you can glean the fruits of Hatha Yoga. For guidance in alignment seek out an experienced Iyengar teacher. For help with *vinyasa* and the *bandhas*, find an experienced Ashtanga Vinyasa Yoga teacher. For help with *Vinyasa Krama*, find a Vinniyoga teacher. However, do not allow the occasional prejudices of teachers of one style to undermine your confidence in the techniques emphasized by other styles. Ultimately, however, you must find your own way, and your own style of practice which suits you in all the changing circumstances and moods of your life.

The Background of Dynamic Yoga

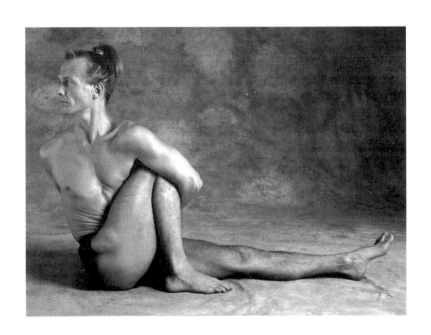

THE BENEFITS OF DYNAMIC YOGA

Dynamic Yoga has something for everyone. It is not only for those who are physically fit, or spiritually inclined. Its effects are so varied, comprehensive and far-reaching that it would be hard to find someone for whom it could offer nothing.

Superficially it is a superlative form of exercise. Unlike most forms of exercise, Dynamic Yoga offers the full range of fitness benefits. It not only develops flexibility, but also strength, stamina and vitality. The gentle stretching action involved in each yoga posture promotes a gradual, safe increase in the flexibility of the whole body. There are hundreds of yoga postures which between them develop flexibility in every single muscle. A flexibility developed gradually and safely. As a result of the careful and precise use of the body in the postures, overstretching is rare.

Dynamic Yoga promotes both cardiovascular and muscular stamina. Cardiovascular stamina is developed through the continuity of action: muscular stamina through sustaining the action of the muscles while holding the postures. Dynamic Yoga is not, however, intentionally aerobic. While initially it will create an increase in heart rate at certain points, eventually this will no longer occur. That it is doing so indicates a lack of fitness and/or difficulty in doing the poses or maintaining the continuity. As your fitness develops, this will happen less. Eventually your pulse will slow down and stay slow. Until this happens it is important to use the finishing inversions and sitting poses to allow the heartbeat to slow down at its own pace.

Muscular stamina is one kind of muscular strength, deeper and more beneficial than that of muscular power. Both muscular power and stamina are developed through the dynamic connectivity of the practice. The lengthening, as opposed to contracting, action of the muscles, however, means that deep strength is developed with much less muscle bulking. The muscle use demanded by Hatha Yoga increases the efficiency of the muscle fibres, rather than simply enlarging them. So the body becomes toned without necessarily becoming larger. Although it will appear to do so due to increased definiton.

One of the first things you will notice, if you practise with care and attention, is a feeling of deep but alert relaxation when you have finished. However, for those people who are residually tired, but who mask that fact with activity and stimulants, there will be a feeling of tiredness. This will pass after a while. Until it does, listen to it, and respect it. Take time to rest in your life. Do not expect your practice to work miracles in the face of a debilitating lifestyle. Use it to help you change your habits so that your whole life, or as much as possible, is nurturing and healing you. With time and consistent practice the relaxation you feel at the end of a session will infuse your life. You will become more and more relaxed within your everyday activities, and within yourself.

The increased circulation resulting from movement and efficient muscle use tones the whole body. The muscles, joints, internal organs, connective tissues and skin are bathed in a continuous flow of fresh blood. This not only brings nutrients to the cells, but helps to purify them of toxic wastes. The heat produced by the practice furthers this purification by opening the cellular tissues to enhance release of toxins. This means that the whole body is cleansed and nourished more efficiently. This in turns optimizes not only the condition of the various parts of the body, but also their functioning. Thereby the respiratory, digestive, circulatory, endocrine, immune and reproductive systems all benefit. In this way your practice will improve your health. With improved health comes increased vitality, enthusiasm and appreciation of life.

This in turn will have a cosmetic effect. As circulation improves so too will skin tone and skin quality. This is further enhanced by the vitality of the internal organs, especially the liver and kidneys, in keeping the body healthy and vital. One of the most striking signs of a seasoned hatha yogin is soft, smooth, shining skin. It is this and the effect of overall body tone on posture that often makes them look much younger than they are. The same vibrant quality conferred on the skin can be seen in the eyes also.

Hatha Yoga affects the mind as much as the body. It improves concentration, increases alertness, precipitates perceptual and rational clarity, cultivates calmness, develops equanimity, instils confidence and nourishes contentment. These benefits all depend on presence of mind during practice.

But Hatha Yoga goes deeper than the mind, penetrating to the core of our being. It is truly a soul-food of unparalleled value. If approached openly, without ambition and pride, specific objectives, predetermined ideals or wishful thinking, it will foster profound self-knowledge. It will also inspire deep self-acceptance, and provide continuous self-validation and self-empowerment. In short: self-love. A love that spills out from itself into a genuine compassion for and interest in all beings and phenomena. This compassion expresses itself in a natural and spontaneous generosity, and an easy, sympathetic humour.

More fertile soil for the flowering of happiness could hardly be found.

3

THE CONTEXT OF DYNAMIC YOGA

Yoga

Yoga is an ocean fed by many rivers, each one fed by many, many streams. The ocean is the ocean, and once there the traces of the rivers that lead to it dissolve. The rivers that lead to the ocean of yoga differ in their courses, but share their destination. It is only when still in the flow of the river that these differences have any significance. Each of these rivers is fed by many streams and rivulets. The range of techniques and tools of yoga is endless and impossible to enumerate or classify exhaustively. Historically there have been five main branches of yoga: *Raja Yoga*, the Royal Path, with emphasis on meditation; *Jnana Yoga*, The Path of Wisdom, with emphasis on self-enquiry; *Hatha Yoga*, The Path of Energy, with emphasis on energetic balancing; *Bhakti Yoga*, The Path of Devotion, with emphasis on worship; *Karma Yoga*, The Path of Action, with emphasis on service.

However, the deeper one goes into any path, the more it reveals and resembles the others in effect, if not in method. The distinctions between them are mostly of emphasis and approach. These differences take into account the broad spectrum of human inclination and aptitude, thereby permitting greater access to the ocean of yoga.

The ocean of yoga represents the highest ideal and attainment of the human being. However it is not a philosophical phenomenon, but an experiential one. In essence it is the undiluted experience of the full potential of human existence. This experience, or state of being, is not exclusive to Yoga. It is accessible by many other spiritual practices from other cultures, East and West. It has been given many names to describe it: all inadequate and partial; but each giving a sense of it from a particular angle. Liberation: freedom from bondage. Emancipation: freedom from the self.

Enlightenment: freedom from delusion. Salvation: freedom from suffering. Self-realization: freedom from the ego.

The word *yoga* itself implies all of these meanings. It is a state of being in which all apparent opposites, distinctions and states are reconciled experientially and ontologically in a state of unity. The word yoga means union. This means not only union of the parts with each other, but also with the whole. Therein we are able to live without fragmentation, or inner conflict. We are able to embrace our whole being from the surface to the depths. We encompass both our transient limitations and our perennial limitlessness. We express through our individuality the wholeness of which we are a momentary fleeting expression. We honour and live from, by and within our true nature. This is the key to a life of peace and contentment.

Hatha Yoga

Hatha Yoga approaches this in a very definite way. It uses all the available aspects of the human being to access the subtle, elusive inner nature of being human. It uses the anatomical, physiological, neural, energetic, perceptual, emotional, rational and intuitive aspects of our being to access our spiritual nature. This is because they are not distinct from it but particular, limited expressions of it. By accessing them fully, integrating and harmonizing them, our latent potential is released, our true nature revealed.

While the ultimate aim of yoga may be profound and daunting, it is far from being irrelevant. Our spiritual nature is not distinct from our social, psychological or animal natures. It is the source and sustenance of them, they the agents and signposts to it. To engage in the process of yoga is not about turning our back on our conditioned selves. Quite the reverse. It involves encountering, acknowledging and accepting ourselves just as we are. To reveal and express what we are in the deepest sense, our true nature, we must learn first to reveal and express what we are on all the other levels of our being.

Yoga is not a process of denial, but revelation. Nor is it a process of creation. Our true, spiritual nature exists. Our imagination, intelligence, enthusiasm and energy, however potent, are not capable of such a creative act: that is the domain of God. All that we can do is clarify its existence, through the practice of yoga; and then honour it in the living of our lives. This is what it means to be holy: to be whole. To live from the wholeness of our human being. This is the state of yoga.

While Hatha Yoga is a river in itself, it is one that has generated many rivulets: the different schools of yoga which all have their own distinct styles. These differences are mainly of emphasis. What they all have in common is the use of the physical body, especially through the yoga postures, known as *Asana*. Their distinctions arise because life is not a monotone. It is a symphony of infinite variety: a tapestry of energetic interweaving that is constantly changing. Interpreting this pattern has led to many symbolic representations of it. One of the simplest, and most pragmatic, is that of the five elements of the natural world.

The Five Elements

One of the most effective ways to grasp the dynamic of life and of yoga is by considering the energetic relationship between the five elements or energies of nature. These five energies, which

5

underlie the five technical processes of the Hatha Yoga method, are fundamental to all processes, situations, events and phenomena. They are symbolically defined as the five elements of the natural world: earth, water, fire, air and space.

They represent the context and the four stages of manifestation. *Space* represents the context of existence, traditionally known as consciousness. *Air* represents the gaseous level of existence, where distinct energies come into play. *Fire* represents the plasmic level, where energies meet, engage and transform. *Water* represents the liquid level of existence, where energies are becoming more focused, more stable, more defined. *Earth* represents the solid level where objects are formed by virtue of stable duration in time and space.

The symbolic representations of these states are useful to us because they are familiar. We have all been interacting with earth, water, fire and air in their many forms since conception. All within the context, not only of physical space, but also awareness, consciousness.

The Element of Space

Space is the primary element within which the four secondary elements emerge and operate. It is the context within which the others interact. Space qualities are immediacy, emptiness, directness, freedom and being. Its fundamental expression is consciousness or awareness, and it is embodied in the technique of *drushti*: focused, directed attention. It leads to a direct and deep awareness of that which is occurring, free from imagination, assumption, projection and expectation. Space is the matrix within which the other elements dance. Its arena is everywhere, its source is consciousness, its medium awareness, and its control concentration. The superficial application of space is sustained concentration. The subtle application of space is surrender of intention. Establishing space requires the utilization of restraint; the sign of its presence is the opposite, freedom.

The Element of Earth

Earth is the fundamental secondary element. Earth qualities are stability, firmness, maintaining, grounding and doing. Its fundamental expression is form, or structure, and it is embodied in the technique of *asana*. Earth is cultivated and expressed by establishing structural integrity in the body. This is done by practising *Asana* according to the principles of alignment (*asana*). The arena of earth is the spine, its source is the foundation of the body, its medium the muscles, and its control the pelvis. The superficial application of earth is to approach alignment in a linear manner, losing oneself in the detail. The subtle application is an intuitive approach, whereby the energy of opposition is utilized to activate emptiness. Establishing earth requires the utilization of pressure; the sign of its presence is the opposite, emptiness.

The Element of Water

Water qualities are softness, fluidity, adaptability, power and feeling. The fundamental expression of water is deliberate movement, and it is embodied in the technique of entering and leaving, arriving and departing: *vinyasa*. Water is cultivated and expressed by learning to move effortlessly, softly and fluidly into, out of and between *Asana*. It is supported by repetition, and expressed in synchronicity between breath and body movement. The arena of water is the pelvis, its source the ball of the foot, its medium the bones, and its control the joints. The superficial application of water is to allow complete passivity into the muscular system, reducing *Asana* to stretch. The subtle application is to find the exact synchronization of body movement and breathing. Establishing water requires the utilization of delicacy; the sign of its presence is its opposite, power.

The Element of Fire

Fire qualities are transformation, suddenness, intensity, radiance and inspiration. The fundamental expression of fire is action, bringing about change, and it is embodied in the technique of *bandha*. Fire is cultivated and expressed through the application of *Uddiyana*, *Mula* and *Jalandharabandha*. The focus of this process is *Uddiyanan bandha*. The arena of fire is the abdomen, its source the solar plexus, its medium the *nadis*, and its control the throat. The superficial application of fire is to generate heat through momentum. The subtle application is to generate heat through *Uddiyanabandha*, while using *Jalandhara* and *Mulabandha* to transform and redirect it. Establishing fire requires the utilization of subtlety; the sign of its presence is its opposite, radiance.

The Element of Air

Air qualities are opening, expansion, lightness, grace, and thinking. The fundamental expression of air is spaciousness, lack of restriction, and it is embodied in the technique of *pranayama*. Air is cultivated and expressed by creating space in the joints and organs, particularly the lungs. The arena of air is the thorax, its source is the throat, its medium the skin (including the nerves), and its control the limbs. The superficial application of air is to develop the capacity to overcome the effect of gravity on the physical body. The subtle application is to free the breath from the limitations of physical and mental tension. Establishing air requires the utilization of movement; the sign of its presence is its opposite, stillness.

The Five Techniques

Hatha Yoga has a very precise set of tools for bringing us deeply in touch with our true nature through the body. They are the five practical techniques, which together constitute the method of Hatha Yoga. Each one of these techniques embodies and expresses one of the energetic qualities of the five elements. In order for yoga practice to be balanced, and access its depths, all these energies must be present and balanced. Together they create an energetic model of the full potential of life. This allows each of the natural energies, and Hatha Yoga techniques, to support all of the others. This not only deepens their effectiveness, but also prevents imbalance between the five energies. The wheel of Hatha Yoga has five major spokes. Its effectiveness depends upon the presence of them all. If one or more are missing the wheel will not roll true, and is susceptible to damage. If one is emphasized at the expense of the others, the same is also true.

Drushti

As far as the practice of Hatha Yoga is concerned, Space represents freedom: the ability to act at will in any manner and direction. It is embodied in *drushti*. *Drushti* is directed attention, in which the energy of awareness is focused on a specific object, process, situation or phenomenon. The process of focusing awareness completely in this way is the essence of spiritual practice, and therefore of yoga. Focusing on the quality of attention is the space aspect of practice.

Asana

Earth represents stability: the ability to maintain structural integrity under stress. It is embodied in *asana*. *Asana* is easy stability in the physical structure, in which each part of the body is aligned with the others to support the whole effortlessly. By stabilizing the body, our mind also begins to stabilize and quieten. Focusing on structure, utilizing the principles of alignment, is the earth aspect of practice.

Vinyasa

Water represents fluidity: harmonious, effortless movement. It is embodied in *vinyasa*. *Vinyasa* is the manner of entering, leaving and joining postures:

the moving aspect of practice. These movements are always done in harmony with the breathing. Focusing on fluidity, utilizing breath body synchronization in entering and leaving a pose, is the water aspect of practice.

Bandha

Fire represents transformation: the process of energetic change that leads to purification. It is embodied in *bandha*. The *Bandhas* are muscular and energetic adjustments that transform our internal energies. By bringing them to a deeper harmony the mind is further quietened. Focusing on transforming and directing energy, is the fire aspect of practice.

Pranayama

Air represents mobility: the ability to move freely, lightly and effortlessly. It is embodied in *pranayama*. *Pranayama* is the process of refining the quality of our breathing. By refining our breath it becomes, slow, smooth, soft and effortless: these qualities then further enhance the quietening of the mind. Focusing on the quality of the breath is the air aspect of practice.

In short, *drushti* is the quality of our awareness, *asana* the quality of our posture, *vinyasa* the quality of our movement, *bandha* the quality of our energy, and *pranayama* the quality of our breathing. It is the quality of these things, not the quantity, that matters in yoga. All of them can be either overemphasized or neglected. Overemphasis on space leads to withdrawal; neglect to anxiety. Overemphasis on earth leads to rigidity; neglect leads to weakness. Overemphasis on water leads to fragility; neglect to hardness. Overemphasis on fire leads to depletion; neglect to dullness. Overemphasis on air leads to instability; neglect to heaviness.

Balanced application of the five techniques of *drushti, asana, vinyasa, bandha* and *pranayama,*

brings about a nurturing balance between the five elements. Only then can the effects of each technique, or presence of each element or energy, lead to its fruition. When our practice is balanced we manifest stability, adaptability, radiance, grace and directness. As these qualities mature in us they allow us to let go more and more of the structures within which we have been hiding ourselves from our true potential. The Five Techniques are explained in practical detail in Part II of this book.

Styles of Hatha Yoga

Ashtanga Vinyasa Yoga

Ashtanga Vinyasa Yoga is a Hatha Yoga system, developed by K. Pattabhi Jois at the behest of Krishnamacharya. It is directly based on the teachings of the Yoga Korunta, adapted to be practicable for citizens of the modern world. It is not strictly a style of yoga but a presentation of Classical Hatha Yoga. However, conscious awareness of the energies of the five elements is often lost in the contemporary teaching milieu. Ashtanga Vinyasa Yoga can be approached in a partial way: overemphasizing one or other aspect of the practice at the expense of the others. This might be heat and fluidity at the expense of alignment. Or it might be strength and flexibility at the expense of sensitivity. This sometimes results in imbalance that does not represent the intrinsic completeness of the system.

Iyengar Yoga

Iyengar Yoga emphasizes alignment, especially through the use of the standing poses, which initiate the Yoga Korunta sequences. This emphasis ensures that the unusual use of the body demanded by *Asana* is not harmful. It respects the laws of structural anatomy, movement and energetics. In order to clarify and ripen this process it sometimes neglects other aspects of Hatha Yoga, the *bandhas*

8

and *vinyasa* in particular. However, a deep familiarity with alignment, *vinyasa* and the *bandhas*, shows that this is not a phenomenon of omission, but emphasis. For if *vinyasa* is the art of moving systematically from one *Asana* to another, the study of alignment includes this in the rigorous precision with which one establishes and releases *Asana*. If *bandha* is the art of adjusting the energetic core of the body, the study of alignment includes this in the precise detail with which one adjusts each part of the body in *Asana*.

Vinniyoga

Vinniyoga emphasizes step by step progression towards a goal (*vinyasa krama*), using the breath as a key and a guide. This allows for particular emphasis on remaining relaxed and sensitive to what one is doing, but sometimes neglects the subtleties of both alignment and the *bandhas*. However, a profound study of *vinyasa krama*, in posture sequencing and the sequential activation of internal adjustments, will reveal the principles of alignment and the subtleties of the *bandhas*.

Power Yoga

Power Yoga emphasizes fluidity and heat, using continuity to support them both. This allows for an intense deepening of concentration and internalization as a result of the challenge and momentum of the practice. However, the emphasis on continuity can lead to a loss of subtlety. On the other hand, if approached openly, without ambition, it can lead to deeply internalized awareness. This awareness then becomes the source of the subtleties of alignment, *vinyasa*, *bandhas* and breathing.

Dynamic Yoga

Dynamic Yoga can be seen and used as a safe, effective stepping stone to the traditional Ashtanga Vinyasa practice. This is because it clarifies each of the technical aspects of Hatha Yoga and integrates them all in the Classical way, but in a modified format. It can also be used as a way to unify the teaching methods of Iyengar Yoga, Vinniyoga and Power Yoga.

Unexpectedly, perhaps, the key to the practice of Hatha Yoga is not so much the technical emphasis, but the attitude and intention of the teacher and the student. The experiential fact is that the different technical aspects of Hatha Yoga are not separate from each other. A profound study of any one of them will lead an open-minded student to all of the others. Therefore the so-called different styles of Hatha Yoga are not absolutely distinct from each other. They complement and even support each other. Hatha Yoga is like a diamond. Although its different facets face in different directions, they support each other, while both containing and leading to its inner sanctum: self-realization. To reach this sanctum we need safety and subtlety (Iyengar Yoga), softness and sensitivity (Vinniyoga), continuity and heat (Ashtanga Vinyasa Yoga), concentration and internalization (Power Yoga), all together. Then we have Hatha Yoga. This is the approach of Dynamic Yoga.

HOW YOGA WORKS

Hatha Yoga as Relaxation

Yoga is a practical method for untapping our hidden and latent potential. It uses the five techniques of *asana*, *vinyasa*, *bandha*, *pranayama* and *drushti* to bring about a state of profound relaxation. This relaxed state is one of vibrant and alert harmony, in which all of the different aspects of our being are integrated and accessible. It emerges once we are completely free from any residual tension. It begins to emerge as soon as we begin the process of releasing the residual tension we carry within us. This tension is so deeply embedded that we are often unaware of its existence. Though it hinders us, we may not know that because we never were, or cannot remember being, without it. So, Hatha Yoga is not simply a matter of relieving us from tensions that disturb us. It can release us completely from all patterns of holding and stagnation down to the deepest, unconscious levels of our being.

All the restrictive patterns of habituated tension that inhibit us are the result of past experience. Intrusive, threatening experiences, of whatever kind, tend to be met by resistance. This is a protective mechanism. However it often backfires in the long term. We react to these intrusions by tightening and hardening: both our bodies and our minds. By doing so we render the intrusion less immediately painful. Unfortunately, however, the effect of the tightening is to solidify muscles and other cells, around the energetic impetus of the intrusion. This solidification buries the energy of the intrusion, and we do not have to face its pain. But it remains inside us: locked in by immobile muscle fibres, blocked veins and capillaries, dammed nerve pathways and dormant synapses. So our unprocessed past remains imposed upon the present. Where it serves only to restrict us, and limit our lives. Yoga can release us from this process. If it is done with sensitivity and awareness. If done absentmindedly or violently it can reinforce this process further. By approaching our practice from the balanced perspective of all the elements of *asana*, *vinyasa*, *bandha*, *pranayama* and *drushti*, we are more likely to free ourselves of it.

Hatha Yoga, then, is not relaxation in a superficial sense. It is more than covering up, or avoiding uncomfortable feelings. If that were all it offered, easier to have a glass of wine, a massage and a hot bath. Hatha Yoga goes much deeper than that. It challenges, reveals and releases our embodied tension. In doing so it releases our full potential. It undertakes this challenge in a precise and systematic manner. There is nothing haphazard or chancy about it. Accurate repeated application of the techniques will elicit specific, predictable results. Inaccurate application will not. The result is a deep sense of relaxation and freedom within one's self. This freedom expresses itself as a grateful, appreciative, compassionate enthusiasm for life and living.

Asana as Relaxation

The basic method is the use of very specific physical postures. This foundation is then built on through the use of the other techniques that are used within it. In fact, without these other techniques being applied, Hatha Yoga is little more than gymnastics. Posture becomes *Asana* through the use of *asana*, *vinyasa*, *bandha*, *pranayama* and *drushti*. Only then can it deliver the full harvest of yoga.

There are hundreds of postures. This has to be the case, in order to penetrate the complex and subtle depths of our neuromuscular system. The more simple postures work more superficially, the more complex more deeply. There is no point in trying to master the more complex ones before the more superficial tensions have been released by the more simple *Asana*. While we might be able, through strength or flexibility, determination or relentlessness, to attain the shape of the pose, it will be at the price of freedom. We will simply be imposing new patterns of force, hardness and tension on old. Whereas, in fact, we must work the other way: layer by layer, stripping away the armour that we have collected throughout our lives.

Every muscle, every organ, joint and nerve is likely to be impregnated, more or less, with some kind of tension. Everyone has their own particular pattern. But we almost all of us suffer from restricted functioning of most of our bodies. Hardness in the muscles, tightness in the joints, dullness in the nerves, stagnation in the capillaries and veins, all combine to limit our range of physical, perceptual, emotional and intuitive responsiveness. In order to make available that responsiveness, we must dissolve the restricting tensions.

Asana challenges the muscles and joints to access their full potential. When that potential is realized blood and nerve impulses can flow freely. Each *Asana* challenges a different network of cells in muscles, tendons, ligaments and organs. One by one they work systematically into every part of the body, and every possible functional relationship between each part of the body. To master a specific *Asana* means to release a specific pattern of neuromuscular relationships from all tension. It also means to supply certain muscles, ganglia, glands and organs with oxygen, glucose, minerals and energy through the blood flow. To release even one of these patterns takes time and constant, consistent repetition. Constant means repeating

11

the actions of the *Asana*, including *asana*, *vinyasa*, *bandha*, *pranayama* and *drushti* over and over again. If there is discontinuity in this repetition the old pattern will reassert itself over the loosening effect of the *Asana*. Consistent means to activate the *Asana* always in the same manner, involving the correct, judicious use of *asana*, *vinyasa*, *bandha*, *pranayama* and *drushti*.

As *Asana* begin to release us from tension something very important is revealed. This is that the body and mind cannot be functionally separated. What we find is that each area of physical resistance, (tension, stagnation, dullness, hardness, weakness, irritation) embodies an emotional pattern. When the habituated, physical pattern begins to be released the emotional pattern begins to emerge. This means that *Asana* can, and inevitably will, bring about emotional release. This very important process can also be hindered by our practice, however. If we do not apply all the techniques, perhaps concerned only with alignment, developing heat or powerful breathing, we can easily override this process and force the emotional pattern deeper. The postures must be approached with the deliberation of *asana* (alignment), the fluidity of *vinyasa*, the subtlety of *bandha*, the rhythm of *pranayama*, and the attentiveness of *drushti*. Then the underlying emotional pattern that was hidden by the physical pattern will be challenged and released.

Making Efforts to Relax

Before this can be done, of course, the *Asana* has to be learned. This is not a matter of just being told or shown how it is done. It is a case of working patiently and gradually into each of the individual areas of resistance within the overall pattern of each *Asana*. Once each of the individual areas involved has been released, then they have to be integrated. Once this has occurred, we can enter

the second stage of *Asana*, where it takes on its nurturing, integrative aspect. In this stage the specific effect of each *Asana* on our physical, energetic and mental structure is absorbed. By holding *Asana* at this stage deep transformation of body, energy and mind occurs. This is a process of opening, revealing, harmonizing and releasing, that brings us more fully to ourselves. No longer held by limiting restrictions the energy of life can flow through us freely. Then it can wash away the dross left over in our systems, and permit the flowering of our full potential.

So, there are two stages to *Asana*. The first is active, corrective, piecemeal, and varies in its specific application from individual to individual. It involves breaking down old patterns of restriction. The second is passive, nourishing, integrative, and is universal in application. It involves releasing our universal blueprint of integration. Both stages take time to master. Mastery requires the full support of all the techniques of *asana*, *vinyasa*, *bandha*, *pranayama* and *drushti*.

The first stage, however, is crucial to the relaxation process. If we are strong, flexible and determined, we can, at least in the short term, impose the shape of *Asana* on our muscles. We can force ourselves into the pose, through heat, force, determination, anxiety, desperation or a combination thereof. This is not *Asana*. The underlying physical resistances, and their deeper emotional wounds, are not released. They are simply momentarily put aside. If we do this day after day, we can convince ourselves, on the basis of rapid physical progress on our mats, that we have accomplished something. But, the real test is when we step off the mat. Is our life any more free from the dissonance and conflict that we can cause through our actions? Are we living out a deeper, clearer understanding of our thoughts, our feelings, our actions and our impact on others? Or are we simply getting stronger and stronger, more and more flexible, more and more pleased with our insular selves?

The first, therapeutic, stage is a prerequisite for the second. Too often students, and even teachers, try to bypass the crucial first stage. They try to impose an imitation of integration on their intrinsic limitations. Being forceful is one way of doing this – a way that is often encouraged on the basis of the idea that Hatha Yoga is supposed to be the yoga of force. So it is, but not that kind of force. It does not mean force as aggression, but force as energy. Another, opposite, way that this is done is always to seek out the line of least resistance, avoiding the limitations imposed by tension, by turning away from them. Neither of these approaches leads to the inner sanctum of yoga. To reach the stage of integration, all the parts involved must be released from their restrictions. Then they can be freely integrated, and *Asana*, having delivered its superficial fruit (relaxation), can deliver its deeper fruit (freedom from the swing of opposites).

This two-stage process applies equally to patterns of tension that restrict our breath, and those that define our mind. Our breathing and our minds are no less locked into restrictive patterns of habituated tension than our bodies. The natural, free, potent rhythm of breathing is inhibited by tensions that restrict the respiratory muscles. These muscles are located mainly in the trunk and throat. Therefore their tensions embody trauma associated with safety, trust and communication. This in itself makes it especially difficult to release these muscles and to free our breathing. The memories underlying the physical tension are so raw and threatening that we are afraid to release them. Yet, the paradox is, that it is not releasing these traumatic traces that hurts, but resisting that release. Holding on to them creates discomfort in the form of tension and anxiety. We deal with it by slipping it below the threshold of our awareness. *Pranayama* in *Asana* reverses this process, bringing them up. As we become conscious of the pain of the physical tension, we can still continue resisting the overall pattern: this is what hurts. When we

stop resisting, and let go into the tension, it simply dissolves, the underlying emotional pattern is set free, and we feel immediately released. Then, and only then, when all the underlying emotional residues have been released, can our lungs inhale and exhale freely. Then the second stage, which depends on the first stage of emotional relaxation, is embarked on. In this stage the breath gradually establishes its own, free, unrestricted rhythms. As we stay with these rhythms, accommodating and enhancing them through the application of our attentive awareness, they become more and more deeply harmonious. This profound harmonious quality directly affects the mind in like manner. We become deeply tranquil, calm, lucid and clear. Into that calm clarity emerge the underlying patterns of our minds.

Pranayama brings about a state of meditation: a harmonizing, clarifying of our mental processes. Here, again, the two-stage process occurs. Here again the resistance to the first stage is immense. Not because of fear of pain this time, but rather fear of uncertainty. Into the clear quiet of our minds come the habitual patterns of our thoughts. Because of the lucid, tranquil quality of the mind, its contents are revealed in a way that they normally are not. Instead of certain thoughts, whether memories, perceptual reactions or simply habits, leading automatically to unintentional chains of associative thoughts, feelings or actions, we notice them entering our mind. We are able to see them simply as thoughts momentarily arising, rather than as signs of our self that we are compelled to indulge or express.

When we find that certain patterns of thought, certain themes, stories, dramas, are repetitive we know that we have found a restrictive pattern of tension in the mind. To release ourselves from this pattern we must challenge it with the light of our awareness. Just as we do physical tensions. Not resisting or restricting our thoughts, nor imposing any preferred thoughts. Simply addressing ourselves to what is there: clarifying it, and embracing the change that comes with illuminating a habituated, unconscious process. This is a life-long process. One that addresses the very deepest layers of tension that we embody. As we release these subtle tensions from both mind and body we begin to be able to face life fearlessly, no longer needing to cling to the certainty of the known. Then the second, integrative stage of meditation, which depends on the first stage of deep psychological relaxation, can develop. It is here that the deepest, richest potential of our true nature comes to light. Once we have systematically released ourselves from physical, emotional and psychological tension.

It is only too easy to overlook the first of these two stages, pretending that relaxation and integration can come without effort. It is equally easy to neglect the second, by moving on from one posture to another as soon as one can do it. Either of these omissions considerably diminishes the potency of Hatha Yoga. And while we may well gain some limited physical, emotional and psychological freedoms and powers, compared to the spiritual freedom that is available they are trivial, and ultimately unsatisfying. To access this spiritual gift, we have to make constant consistent effort in the first stage, and we have to spend time in the quiet, assimilative second stage of each process. In the first stage *asana* and *vinyasa* are particularly important. In the second, *bandha* and *pranayama*. *Drushti*, or directed attention, is crucial to both.

While these two stages are an ongoing characteristic of practice at all levels, they are also expressed in the traditional practice format (*sadhana*). This can be divided into two parts. The first is the dynamic stage, expressing the active, creative energy of the solar principle Ha. The second is the passive stage, expressing the passive, receptive energy of the lunar principle Tha. Once the sequence of poses is complete, and before lying in *Savasana*, we finish in a sitting position:

traditionally the full Lotus. The traditional sitting practice of *Pranayama* then focuses on refining and releasing the breath, while the body is held still in a posture that maximizes freedom in the ribcage. This release is brought about through directed attention. Eventually, when freedom of the breath has brought stillness to the mind, we let go of our breath and enter into meditation.

To the extent that we have managed to release our breath, our mind will be still. At this point, we allow our breath, our energy, our posture and our awareness to settle freely into themselves. This is a matter of letting go. If this is not to be simply a physical and mental collapse we must first have utilized the potential of the first dynamic stage to release us from restricting limitations. With practice this will happen more and more. The two stages of *Asana* are then reflected in the two stages of *sadhana*. First activity to release our habitual limitations, then stillness to facilitate ripening of our latent potential. This is the spiritual gift of Hatha Yoga: a release of ourselves to ourselves so profound and complete as to be a rebirth.

The Edge

In order to deliver this priceless gift Hatha Yoga has to bring us constantly to the very limits of our self. This may be in terms of body or mind. It must bring us to our edge. At the point of balance between too much and not enough is our edge. Physically this means utilizing the full capacity of our bodies in this moment. It means neither going too far, nor not going far enough. To find this balance requires an honest sensitivity that can be developed through practice. Mentally it means being willing to stay in the pose long enough for it to yield its fruit. It means not succumbing to haste, impetuousness, distraction, boredom, fear or uncertainty. Instead we must develop and use a clear awareness of what is actually happening. Then coming out of a pose will happen spontaneously and effortlessly. It is equally possible to overstay our welcome in a pose. This can happen easily if we miss our edge. If we do this our energy begins to ebb, our awareness to dissipate. There is a perfect moment to move on. By cultivating honest sensitivity we can learn to respond to that moment, and move on out of the pose. This is not helped by timing our stay in a pose, either by the clock, our breath or our heartbeat. In the beginning, however, such measures may be necessary. But we should not become attached to them. It is of the essence of yoga to go beyond quantitative measurement into the timeless.

By not using enough effort we shortchange ourselves. By using too much we violate ourselves. In between is the edge. The edge is an exhilarating place. But it can be scary. We all know what it feels like to stand at the edge of a cliff. In yoga, it is here, at the edge of the cliff that the fertility lies. Through practice we must learn to find the edge of ourselves, the edge of the pose. Having found the edge, that is when we hold, we stay, we allow ourselves to become still, receptive. Then we find that the edge moves. We do not have to make it do so. It just does. By reaching our current edge, by utilizing our current capacity to the full, the edge moves, our capacity spontaneously increases. This is how we grow. This is how our practice and our capability mature.

Approaching our practice as an exploration helps us to develop the honest sensitivity that reveals our edge. This means going into each pose simply to find out what is there. To discover our current cocktail of tension, freedom, dullness, vitality, movement, stagnation, etc. To discover, acknowledge, accept and express it: fully. It is the nature of life that that which is able fully to be itself will change. It will either grow, or dissolve. In this way yoga enhances our life: allowing that which retains potential to mature, and that which has peaked to pass.

There is no need for us to impose a predetermined destination on ourselves. This can be difficult. The temptation to be caught by the conceptual description of a pose, or seduced by the capacity of others, is great. But it is not helpful. We are what we are. We will change only according to our current capacity. Any change that we impose on that capacity will not last, and may result in problems. We must be patient, and we must be honest, in our practice and in our lives. We must learn to act from love, not desire. To be willing to find the beauty and the value in what we have, what we are. Rather than overlooking, denying or resenting what we are while chasing something we have heard of or seen. It may not be for us.

In discovering the potential of the edge we learn that force is completely unnecessary in Hatha Yoga. The techniques themselves are pregnant with power. We do not need to add to them with misguided impetuosity and impatience. Force used to push through our current limitations is dangerous. This is not only the risk of overstretch to muscles, tendons and ligaments. It also nourishes the sense of inadequacy that generates the grasping quality that must have more. Moreover it sanctifies the greed in which that grasping manifests. In terms of flexibility it is not as helpful as you might think. It is true that by pushing past your limits you gain length in the muscle fibres. But only momentarily. If you do not maintain that momentum in your practice daily, then the overall effect is one of long-term shortening relative to the stretching achieved. For the mechanical result of overstretch is a compensatory shortening: tightening or increase in tension. If, on the other hand, you respect your edge, and utilize cellular intelligence to release your limitations effortlessly, you will find that you do not need to maintain an intense daily practice to maintain your flexibility. Flexibility gained through intelligence is more permanent than that gained by force.

There is more to the edge than physical capability. More profoundly it is the place where all polarities meet and resolve themselves in each other. It is the space of dissolution, surrender, where self and other unify. It is where our ego blends into our self, our conditioned structure merges into our true nature. This place is extremely scary for ego, which depends on the dualistic separations of self and other, inside and outside, remaining clearly delineated. When we come to the edge everything becomes blurred. This brings up huge amounts of resistance. The ego does not want to be disempowered. But to taste the fruit of yoga this is what we must allow to happen. We must be willing to come to the edge, and to surrender our resistance, to stay there, right on the edge. Then we can enter the timeless space of yoga. This is known as dying in the pose. It is necessary for the fruit of yoga to ripen. It can do so at any time. It is not a question of years and years of practice, and then, maybe, one day, I might, if I work hard, get a glimpse of my true nature, my true state. It is already here. It requires no accomplishment on your part. If you want to know it, to feel it, to be it, you must die to your ego, your sense of yourself as a continuous isolated centre. By coming to the edge in a pose you are given an opportunity to do that, momentarily. You can take it whenever you like. Just let go of the resistance, drop the fear, and feel body and mind dropping away from what they had been obscuring.

Of course, this dying cannot occur if we try to push through our edge to get more movement, or to spend more time. It is not a question of space or time. Then we just reinforce our ego, push away the opportunity to dissolve our conditioned structure into our true nature. Often we do not realize that this is what we are doing. The power of ego, to subvert anything to maintain itself, is tremendous. Not wanting to become redundant it eggs us on, with the stick and carrot of 'this is not enough, more is better.' Then we remain caught in duality;

where self and other, and all other polarities, remain separate and antagonistic. If however we can stay with the waves of instability that start to rise when we are on the edge we will find out what yoga is about. When we stay right on our edge the challenge to ego makes it waver. As we stay longer the challenge increases. As the challenge increases the ego becomes more and more unstable: finds it harder and harder to maintain its solid, consistent presence. This can be frightening, and as you go further into it, even terrifying. But it is ego, and only ego, that is afraid, terrified. There is more to you than that. If you can overcome this resistance to ego dying, and stay as you are, you will find the other side. The edge will dissolve, and you will experience your true self. Learning to allow this to really happen is the essence of all spiritual practice. Hatha Yoga is designed to give you that opportunity over and over again, in many different ways. Each *Asana* has its own edge. Each edge is a doorway to your true self. It opens by itself, all you have to do is get to the threshold and stay there, resisting the huge impetus to retreat, or the subtle demand to push on through.

Cellular Intelligence

Our mind is not located only in the brain. It exists in every cell of our body. *Asana*, therefore, is not just a question of muscular flexibility and power, and joint mobility. These alone are only the base. The superstructure is the awakening of cellular intelligence. This we bring about through sensitivity, through feeling what we are doing. Directing what we are doing to the most precise degree, to the most subtle level. To awaken the intelligence in each part of the body as we enter each posture. To deepen that intelligence as we hold the posture. And to maintain that intelligence as we leave, and then bring it to the next. It is by awakening and utilizing cellular intelligence that we can move the body without force, and safely, into positions strange and wonderful. Without it the tendency to use potentially dangerous force is tempting. Many postures can be achieved through strength or flexibility, without being *Asana*. Without bringing the benefits of Hatha Yoga. Without this somatic intelligence, yoga is just exotic stretch exercise. It is the combined effect of the five techniques, rather than just the shapes, that awaken this intelligence.

Making Balance

Hatha Yoga is the yoga of balance. This is indicated by the term Hatha. Ha means solar current, energizing principle, creative force. Tha means lunar current, pacifying principle, receptive force. Hatha Yoga is the means whereby these, and all other, opposing forces are brought into balance on every level of our being. This state of balance is one in which opposites lose their conflict, and resolve themselves in each other. In practice there are a number of pairs of opposites that must be well balanced in our practice. If one member of a pair outweighs the other consistently, problems will arise.

ACTION AND STILLNESS
We need to find a balance between activity and rest: between time spent in poses, and time spent moving between them. *Asana* itself is restful, there is therefore no need to rest from the poses. Unless of course we are overdoing them by approaching them superficially in terms of quantity rather than quality. Each *Asana* has a dynamic and a static aspect. The way we move into a pose influences its quality. The way we move out colours its effect. Having taken all the necessary steps to enter a pose as fully as possible, we should then pause, motionless except in our breathing. With practice we will learn to feel how long we need to spend in

stillness. Then we leave. However, this stillness retains a dynamic quality. The adjustments we have made in entering, especially the *bandhas*, need to be maintained. While we are no longer moving in space, we are active internally. While we have physical resistance in the beginning to the challenge of moving, we have a mental resistance to staying still. At various times we will find ourselves resisting one or the other more. We have to listen to this resistance to find out what is behind it. If it is fear or boredom, or laziness, we drop the resistance. If we find it is because our actual capacity, whether mental or physical, is below par, we honour it. Too much action, too much emphasis on the dynamic aspect of practice can lead to exhaustion and biological and energetic depletion. Too much rest in between postures can lead to absentmindedness, superficiality and lack of vitality. Eventually we learn to find the rest within activity, the dynamism of rest. In this way we learn the unity underlying these poles.

STRENGTH AND FLEXIBILITY
Dynamic Yoga offers an equal opportunity to both strength and flexibility. However each individual will choose their own emphasis. Usually, though not always, this will be the emphasis that is easier. If this is the case, however, we will simply be playing into our own imbalance. Rather we should see which way we tend and use our practice to make balance. Strength and flexibility are not just a matter of the muscles. Do we tend to push and bludgeon our way through life, or do we make way too easily in the face of difficulty? Are we strong enough to withstand difficulty? Are we adaptable enough to ride life's waves with a smile? Muscles with a lot of movement can be that way through a lack of stability or resilience in the fibres: this is superficial flexibility. Muscles with the forceful power that comes from bulk lack the efficiency to vary their load-bearing: this is superficial strength. Too much emphasis on developing superficial

strength can hinder flexibility. Too much emphasis on superficial flexibility can diminish deep strength and stability. This applies to our minds as well as our bodies. A truly strong mind is one that can adapt. A flexible mind is one that can cope with anything. Likewise a strong body can accommodate any challenge, a flexible one will not break under any amount of pressure.

WARMING AND COOLING

Hatha Yoga is a fire technique. It generates heat. However, this heat is to be transformed by the *bandhas*. Too much physical heat leads to depletion. Sweat should form a protective, insulating coat on the surface of the body and not drop off profusely. Excessive sweating is a sign of excess liquid in the body, over-exertion or both. By the time we come to the end of our practice, however, the body should be cool. This is facilitated by the finishing sequences incorporating the inversions, sitting postures and *Savasana*. Enough time needs to be spent on them to ensure adequate cooling. If not we can take the fire from our practice into our lives, where it may be neither appropriate nor containable. Hatha Yoga is an intense practice, but if undertaken judiciously results in a coolness of mind and subtlety of movement. Of course, this coolness can also be taken too far. Excessive inversions and sitting can lead to withdrawal and a lack of psychological vitality.

EFFORT AND EASE

The Hatha Yoga techniques require effort. However, it must be considered effort. It should create no strain, no struggle, no tension. A balanced, judicious application of effort gives a sense of effortless ease. This can be seen clearly in the practice of an accomplished Hatha Yogin. We have to find a creative balance between imposition (too much effort) and complacency (too much ease). This involves finding our edge. Once we

develop a sense for our edge we can dance on it experimenting with the effort that is not force, and finding the effortlessness that is not inertia.

ACTION AND MEDITATION

Meditation is not a vacuous trance. It is a clear, comprehending apprehension of that which is, just as it is. It is a vibrant, effortless, encompassing awareness. In Hatha Yoga this is established through activity, not inactivity. The subtle adjustments that we make in establishing *asana*, *vinyasa*, *bandha* and *pranayama* serve to cultivate presence of mind. In order for *Asana* to occur these adjustments cannot be made piecemeal, in a sequential, linear manner. We must learn to activate them simultaneously. When we are able to do this, so that the adjustments occur instantly, we are meditating. We are utilizing a panoramic field of awareness which is equally conscious throughout. The actions that we use, the adjustment we establish, are the lattice upon which we thread the strands of our meditative awareness. Then our body becomes the *mandala* upon which we transform our consciousness from one of selective, dualistic distinctions to that of inclusive, unified identity. We use the adjustments, which involve both mind and body, awareness and activity, to dissolve the distinction between body and mind. Because our mind is the subject, our body the object, we also erase the distinction of subject and object which typifies the fragmentation of consciousness that meditation relieves. Hatha Yoga then, taking the body as its seed, is the way of meditation in action.

Presence of Mind

In your practice be aware of all of these polarities and use them to help you find a balance between the five techniques and elements that brings you to the deepest possible state of relaxation. The key to this whole process is a willingness and ability to come into the present. To make contact with exactly what you are doing right now. To experience exactly how that feels. Without any evasiveness. To do what you are doing totally. To feel what you are feeling honestly and fully. To be what you are without dissimulation or prevarication. Each of the techniques of *asana, vinyasa, bandha, pranayama* and *drushti* assists this process in its own way. Through them we can access the present fully, thereby releasing the past and the future. This absolutely cannot occur if we attempt to impose anything on ourselves. Whether that be a range of movement, a shape, a depth of breathing, a preconceived thought pattern, or whatever. We have to surrender to the present in the form of that which actually is. Not that which we would prefer to have, be or do. This means we must be tolerant and patient of our limitations. This does not mean to be complacently accepting of them. Quite the reverse. We use our tolerance and patience to reveal them to us. Then we challenge them, with *asana, vinyasa, bandha, pranayama* and *drushti.* Not with our arbitrary ideals or unrealistic ambitions.

Imposition is attempting to do that which we are not yet ready or able to do. Challenge is activating our actual potential to the full. There is a world of difference in the effect of imposition and challenge in Hatha Yoga. One takes us deeper and deeper into self-conflict. The other gradually releases us from it.

It has taken us years to develop our own peculiar patterns of restricting tension. It will take time to release them. But it does not have to take as long to dismantle them as it did to establish them. Attention is energy. The energy of focused attention (*drushti*) reinforces and enhances the effect of the other techniques. Progress then can be rapid. If our practice is balanced and judicious, then the more we practise the faster the pace. However, for the effects of our practice to be integrated into the daily rhythm of our lives, we must spend time living. Most significantly, in relationship, of one kind or another, to other human beings. Yoga does not work in isolation, unless you stay isolated. Some time you have to come down the mountain, enter the market place again. Then you will see if your practice has been an imitative imposition, or a genuine liberation.

II

The Techniques of Dynamic Yoga

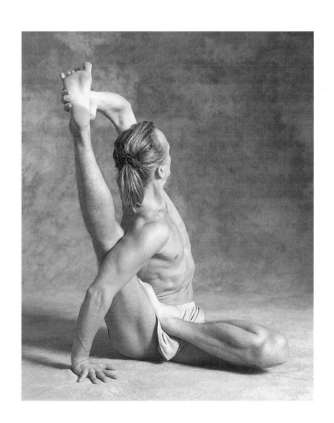

4

DRUSHTI: THE QUALITY OF AWARENESS

The five techniques of the Hatha Yoga method are facets of a single diamond, supporting each other in symbiotic intimacy. This intimacy means than none can flourish or ripen without the others. The manner of entering a posture (*vinyasa*) is bound to facilitate or hinder, more or less, our ability to establish structural equilibrium (*asana*). In order for the core of the body to be energized (*bandha*) accurately, it must be supported by structural equilibrium. When the *bandhas* are fully established their opening and charging of the ribcage spontaneously draws air effortlessly in and releases it effortlessly out (*pranayama*). Directing attentive awareness (*drushti*) to each part of the body to ensure that it is functioning as an integrative part of a harmonious whole underlies the presence of all the other techniques. It must be taken into account then, that conceptual and verbal delineations between *asana, vinyasa, bandha, pranayama* and *drushti* do not mirror the experience of pragmatic reality. While they are five from the outside, from the inside they are one.

Drushti is the context within which the other techniques can occur. Without it they can only remain abstractions, idealized notions that we may think we are expressing, but in fact may not be. Without awareness Hatha Yoga is simply acrobatic exercise. Absentmindedness is the most common hindrance to yoga practice. Presence of mind is its key.

This is most clearly cultivated through the practice of *drushti*. *Drushti* means focusing open, free, full, direct attention on a given place, activity, sensation, quality or vibration. When attention is open it brings with it neither prejudice nor expectation. When attention is free it is not imposed, but establishes itself naturally. When attention is full there is nothing else accommodated by it other than its intended object:

concentration is complete. When attention is direct it is immediate and effortless. When our attentive awareness has all of these qualities it can be called *drushti*. In the meantime, we must be patient and learn through constant repetition.

There are two aspects to *drushti*, quantitative and qualitative. In order for the integrity of *Asana* to be established, each part of the body must take its place, and assume it functions. This includes entering the *Asana* smoothly, effortlessly and in harmony with the breath (*vinyasa*). It also includes establishing lines of force throughout the body so as to establish structural equilibrium (*asana*). It further involves activating the subtle grips that transform the energetics of the pose (*bandhas*). Last, but not least it means ensuring that no force or strain is imposed on the breath (*pranayama*).

In the beginning we are only capable of establishing all of these adjustments of mind and body in a linear, sequential manner. This not only means that it takes time to establish *Asana*, but also that often we lose some adjustments while attending to others. This is an unavoidable part of the learning process. As we mature in our practice, clarification of the intimate relationships that exist between all of these actions allows them to trigger each other simultaneously. Finally they all occur as one. It is when this unitive quality emerges that we are able to dissolve our awareness in the integrity of the pose. When the inner quality of the pose emerges and absorbs our awareness this is *drushti*, or choiceless awareness.

The qualitative aspect of *drushti* permits us to feel the *Asana* as a whole, absorbing and expressing its quality and its nature. This is an inner activity, which has an external mirror. This is the point at which the gaze of our eyes directs itself. Just as our inner gaze is directed to the integrity of the *Asana* itself, our eyes direct themselves to a specific point

which expresses and supports that integrity. In the section presenting instruction in the method of the pose, the external *drushti* gaze point is given as for beginners. This means that a gaze point is given that takes into account the common structural limitations of a body carrying tension.

For example, in Downward Dog (*Adhomukhasvanasana*) you are asked to let your head hang, and gaze towards your legs. The traditional *drushti* is the navel. However, most honest students will have to admit that this they can only do if they arch their backs, bend their legs or drop their shoulders. This is forcing the *drushti* without establishing structural support. The gaze point is then reduced to a conceptual imposition while the integrity of *Asana* is compromised. Whereas the gaze point, when the integrity of the pose is present, is the natural resting point of the eyes. The energy of the pose itself takes the eyes there as a natural expression of itself. The *drushti* is an indication that *Asana*, or meditative awareness with the body as mandala, has occurred. This depends upon each part of the body having taken its place and assumed its function. This is brought about through the adjustments of *asana*, *vinyasa*, *bandha* and *pranayama*.

While the other four pragmatic techniques of Hatha Yoga depend upon *drushti*, so too does *drushti* depend upon them. With attentive awareness the various internal adjustments can be made. As they are made they clarify and deepen our awareness. This further clarity permits more subtle and elusive adjustments. In this way the five techniques provide a self-supporting dynamic that transforms posture into *Asana*.

Within this transformation the distinctions between the five aspects, or elements, begins to blur. Until eventually it becomes clear that they are not separable from each other. Indeed they are just

23

differing manifestations of the same process: *Asana*. In entering a pose with due attention to the breath and the sequential, harmonious activation of various muscle groups (*vinyasa*), alignment (*asana*) is guaranteed. By activating the subtle grips of the *bandhas*, the process of alignment is refined, ripened and energized. By energizing the trunk and the core of the body, the breath is encouraged to flow freely, fully and evenly (*pranayama*). All of this, of course, requires directed attentiveness (*drushti*).

Wherever else our attention is held it must always encompass the core of our body. The core of our body includes the brain, the eyes, ears and tongue, the front and interior of the spine, the area in front of the spine, the pelvic floor and the navel. These areas, collectively known as the core of the body, should remain soft at all times. If the core of the body becomes hard and tight, the posture (no longer *Asana*) will generate tension rather than dissolve it. It will also disturb the rhythm and quality of our breathing. The quality of the core of our body is a vital indicator of the quality of *Asana*. It is far more important than quantity of extension or stretch. The core of our body in its softness should be the centre and source of our awareness (*drushti*), extending itself, with practice, into every cell of the body on the effortless rhythm of our breathing.

Simply speaking, *drushti* is sensitive awareness to that which you are doing. This has two aspects that are vital to every aspect of our practice. First it means bringing your mind to bear exactly on what you are doing. Not doing one thing while thinking another. This actually means learning not even to be thinking about what you are doing. Rather, just be doing it, feeling it. In the beginning we must think before we act. Then we act. Then think again. But we must learn to separate these two processes so that we can act with precision and clarity, without the distraction of thought. Eventually we will learn to trust the intelligence of the body and

will be able to dispense with the thinking process more and more. Then our practice becomes meditation in action.

The second aspect is to feel the effect of what we are doing. Not only at the point of the action itself, but throughout the whole structure of the body and the quality of the mind. We must feel its impact on the functioning of body, breath and mind. We use this feedback to go deeper into the poses by making adjustments according to the four secondary techniques of *asana*, *vinyasa*, *bandha* and *pranayama*. Then through the dynamic created between our attention and our actions, a meditative awareness emerges.

As our practice develops a meditative quality, it is important to spend time sitting quietly at the end of our practice. The dynamic, warming part of Hatha Yoga *Sadhana* has a profound effect on our energetic equilibrium. It shakes and stirs our old patterns. Then the dross begins to surface. We must give it the space to do so. This we do during the passive, cooling part of the practice. But it must be done consciously. We must allow the feelings and thoughts that arise as a result of our 'shakedown' to take the time and the place that they seek. Only then will the underlying tensions, and their unresolved origins, be able to resolve themselves. This resolution occurs in the light of our directed attention: *drushti*.

Drushti has three major qualities: focus, openness, directness. Through focus deep concentration is developed. Through openness detachment is cultivated. Through directness penetration is fostered. All of these qualities are necessary to the resolution of our underlying psychic blocks. Through concentration we develop the stability of mind to cope with the energetic waves of emerging emotional disturbances. Through detachment we develop the clarity to see them for what they are, without having to lose ourselves in them. Through penetration we illuminate them fully, not just as a passing wave,

24

but also in terms of origin, context, implications and consequence. It is this illumination that permits resolution of the emerging structural/energetic/emotional patterns or blocks.

ASANA: THE QUALITY OF FORM

Hatha Yoga is not posturing. There is much more to *Asana* than making a shape in space. It is what is going on inside that shape that is important. The foundation of this is the structural equilibrium established by subtle muscular adjustment: alignment (*asana*). It is alignment (*asana*) that gives posture the grace, stability and ease that characterize *Asana*. It is alignment (*asana*) also that gives *Asana* its therapeutic power: its ability to restructure the anatomical body, and nourish the physiological body. Alignment (*asana*) is the very essence of *Asana*, and without it all the other aspects, of *vinyasa*, *bandha*, *pranayama* and *drushti*, flounder. It must therefore be the practical foundation upon which *Asana* is built and into which the other aspects are integrated.

The basic purpose of alignment is to harmonize the body. This may or may not involve structural perfection. That depends on the capacity available to us in the moment. More importantly it involves harmonizing opposing lines of force. This process, while it may not immediately bring about structural perfection, brings about structural stability. At the same time, it awakens the latent power and intelligence of each cell of the body. Eventually, through consistent repetition, as tension is drawn out of the body cells these lines of force establish deeper and deeper structural harmony and integrity. However, to attempt to impose idealized notions of geometric perfection on the specific realities of our distorted body structures is counterproductive. It not only more deeply entrenches habitual tension, but also often creates new ones. Furthermore it undermines our ability to relate to that which actually exists if we constantly try, from anxious ambition, to impose some notion of desired perfection upon ourselves. If we work with and from our actual limitations and imperfections we will find ourselves approaching so-called perfection effortlessly and inevitably.

In order to support *Asana*, each part of the body must take its place, and assume its functions. Pragmatically this is a process of muscular adjustment. As a result of which, bones move, joints open, the spine and organs change position and shape. Therefore each muscle must be employed precisely in relationship not only to those connected to it, but also those that complement or oppose it. It is a question of establishing balance between the necessary adjustments so that each adjustment supports, rather than hinders structural equilibrium and stability. The key to establishing this balance is to ensure that every line of force that results from a muscular adjustment is met with complementary opposing ones. Because the body is three-dimensional, each line of force is met and supported by more than one opposing force. This also reflects the fact that no muscles exist in isolation. Simply lifting the arms alongside the ears reverberates through the whole musculature. These opposing forces act as limits on each individual adjustment in the various directions of its impact, ensuring that it does not overstep the mark and produce disequilibrium. Their combined effect is to create a series of spirallic momentums in the body that support and complement each other. The lines of force are only straight when seen in isolation, or partially. If we follow their momentum through we find they are all spirallic, and connected to each other spirallically.

Establishing the full range of muscular adjustments throughout the whole body necessary to *Asana* often means bringing life and awareness to habitually dormant cells and muscles. This means that in the beginning the body may not respond. Before the body can obey the mind, new neural pathways must be established between the brain and the muscle, and between the muscle and the brain, and between various parts of the brain, and then back again to the muscle. This takes time. Be patient. Again, consistent repetition is the only way. Somebody can push or pull you into a new position but if the innate intelligence of the required body cells is not awakened by activation of its contextual neural circuitry, then nothing useful to *Asana* will have been learned. Adjusting the body into *Asana* is not simply a matter of overcoming the physical limitations of the muscles. It is more fundamentally one of awakening the somatic intelligence of the entire body. As cellular intelligence begins to awaken, it lends itself to more and more subtle, effective and comprehensive adjustments.

Of all the yoga postures the most important for awakening somatic intelligence are the standing postures. This is not only because they develop the feet and the legs, which are the fundamental supports of our spinal column. Each standing pose requires activity in each part of the body in order for stability to be established. There are no inert areas, and very little passivity. There are so many vital supporting relationships that need to be established in a standing posture in order to maintain equilibrium. In more advanced poses this is not so. The extremes of motion in some parts of the body are compensated for by absolute relaxation of others. The extreme complexity of the lines of force involved in standing postures awakens somatic intelligence thoroughly and deeply. Although this process can be a very lengthy one of many years, overall progress into advanced *Asana* is more rapid, as well as safer, than if the standing poses are not given enough emphasis. This is why each of the Classical Hatha Yoga series begins with a sequence of standing poses. Somatic intelligence, having been awakened in the standing poses, is then available when attempting more advanced and strenuous *Asana* which otherwise require extremes of strength, flexibility or insensitivity.

It is a paradox of *Asana* practice that the more advanced the *Asana* the fewer options one has for erring: error brings immediate problems. In the more basic *Asana*, the options are many, and errors can pass unnoticed to the inexperienced gaze. We either have the capacity, in terms of mobility in the pelvis, back, neck and hamstrings to put a leg behind our neck, or we don't. If we don't and we try to impose the pose on that limitation, we will hurt ourselves, immediately and obviously. In standing poses, error is not so obvious, nor so immediately harmful. We are all capable of standing more or less straight with our feet together, and learning safely to refine this position. Therefore we can safely work within our limitations, and use the standing poses as a secure foundation for the advanced postures.

The accessible complexity of the standing poses contrasts directly with the elusive simplicity of the advanced poses. However, the simplicity of the advanced poses rests entirely on the groundwork established within the complexity of the standing poses. If we have not awakened the intelligence of the legs, pelvis, spine, shoulders and neck, we are likely to hurt ourselves when attempting to put our leg behind our neck. If we have not awakened the intelligence in limbs, hands, feet, pelvis, shoulders and spine, we are likely to hurt ourselves even in simple backbends such as Upwards Dog (*Urdhvamukhasvanasana*). We will not be sensitive to the impulses that tell us where we are blocked, where we are free, when we have reached our safe limit, and how, therefore we have to adjust our movements accordingly in order to achieve our aim.

Alignment (*asana*) is learned about, and established, in the standing poses. If not, the advanced poses can only be done from extremes of strength and flexibility that may not acknowledge, express or nurture the current capacity and structural integrity of the body. This is not *Asana*, but gymnastics or acrobatics, and will not bring

about self-knowledge, self-acceptance or self-validation. Instead, it may bring about pride, attachment to appearances, and subtle internal conflict.

When alignment (*asana*) transforms posture into *Asana*, certain qualities emerge. One is effortless stability. Another is alert ease. Anatomically these depend upon the ability of the muscles to calibrate and stabilize themselves throughout the whole body. In order for the musculature as a whole genuinely to stabilize itself, no single muscle or muscle group must be under any strain or carrying any tension. This takes time to establish. Some muscles need to be strengthened, some need to be relaxed. Some need to be lengthened, some need to be shortened. Some need to be rested, some need to be awakened. All of these complementary adjustments occur naturally as a result of consistently applying the appropriate lines of force throughout the whole body.

The subtle details of alignment are endless, and do not all need to be consciously considered in order for them to come about. The interconnectedness of each part of the body to all other parts ensures that as our practice matures, our sensitivity becomes more subtle and our awareness deepens, many adjustments occur spontaneously, and we become aware of them doing so. To try to master alignment the other way round, by analysing each pose into every detail and trying sequentially to impose them, is like trying to empty the ocean with a spoon. Better we start with an understanding of the basic principles, and take care of overall structural stability. Then as our sensitivity develops and open attention deepens we will be guided by the feedback of our bodies more and more deeply into the pose. Then we do not necessarily consciously initiate exactly what is happening muscle by muscle.

The living human organism, and all its parts, are in continual flux. Therefore no single adjustment can be permanently or absolutely valid. The living dynamic of the body will not happily yield to the static nature of words and concepts. Do not try to force it to do so. Accordingly, this section presents the underlying principles of alignment in some of their more fundamental and necessary applications. It could not hope, nor intends, to be exhaustive. This section is simply designed to offer a firm foundation to guide your mind and body in their own enquiry into and exploration of alignment. The sooner you are able to experience the operation of the principles described at the end of this section, the sooner you will be able to enjoy this fascinating journey solo.

Your reading of the following will be greatly enhanced if you try all of the actions referred to as you go along. While a picture may be worth a thousand words, an action is worth thousands of pictures. Yoga is a practical activity. Trying out all of these actions now will greatly facilitate your practice of the postures. But remember that complete assimilation comes only through repeated practice within the context of the postures.

The Foundation

The most fundamental aspect of alignment is the quality of contact with the floor. This is our support, our foundation. Only if this is stable and even can overall structural stability be established. This means that our full body weight must be spread evenly over the whole foundation. For example, in Downward Dog (*Adhomukhasvanasana*) the hands and feet are the foundation, each being one corner. Each of these corners should carry one quarter of the body weight. Remember that these principles apply holographically. Therefore each of the four corners has four corners which must activate in the same

way. This can be taken to whatever depth your sensitivity allows. From this even foundation the trunk can lift freely upwards, and the spine can release evenly and fully.

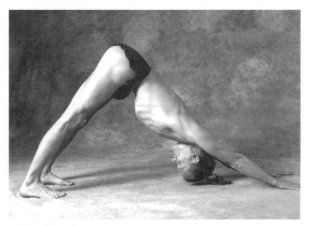

Adhomukhasvanasana

Of course, in the beginning this may not be possible. Perhaps because of stiffness in the lower back, hips or legs, weight cannot be brought evenly onto the feet. Practice of this and the standing postures will eventually make it possible.

In any standing pose in which both feet are on the floor, no matter what spatial relationship they have to each other, they share the body weight equally. So too does each part of the foot. That means weight is spread evenly between the left and right foot; between the balls of the feet and the heels; between the inner edge and the outer edge of the feet. This means that the front, back, inner and outer leg muscles will be equally supported and so can activate evenly, allowing the knee joint to be centred and the head of the thigh bone to rest evenly in the hip socket. This of course depends also on the exact position of the feet, which is indicated in the instructions for each posture.

The body's foundation is not only and always the feet. In Downward Dog it is hands and feet. When the hands are used as part of the foundation, bearing

29

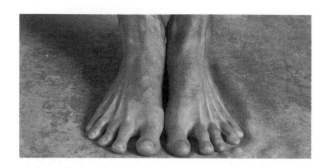

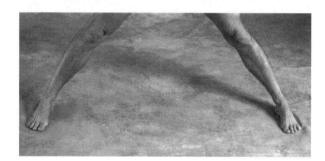

some or all of the body's weight, they must be used in a similar manner. This means that their share of the weight, perhaps all or perhaps half the body weight, must be shared evenly between them, and equally throughout the contact they have with the floor.

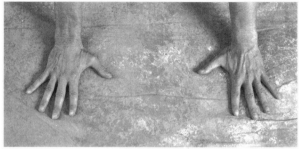

30

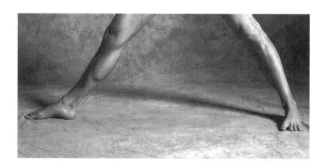

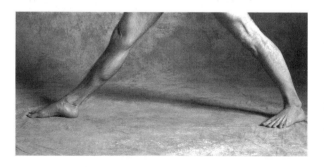

In order for this to be so the palms must be broad, the bases of the fingers spread wide without strain, the fingers long and centred, with even spaces between them, and the heels of the hands in clear contact with the floor. Especial care must be taken, because of the effect of the ball of the thumb, to keep the index finger base on the floor. This should not be at the expense of the heel of the hand or the little finger base. In effect though, maintaining contact with the base of the index finger and the floor becomes the fulcrum of learning to use the hands against the floor. It is from this point that we move in and out of the postures of the *vinyasa*, and those in the middle section of the Sun Salutation.

Other parts of the body can also be our foundation. They should be used according to the same principle of creating an even, stable equilibrium that does not depend on undue strength, force or extreme flexibility. In the Headstand, for example, the foundation is the crown of the head, the outer edge of the wrists and forearm bone, and the flesh of the inner forearm. No strain should be felt in the neck. This requires lift from the shoulders supported by the action of the upper arms, wrists and thumbs.

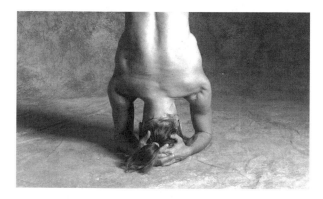

This lift is supported by the even foundation.
Similarly in the Shoulderstand. The foundation is the back of the skull, the back top of the shoulder girdle, the upper arms and the elbows. Weight should not be carried on the vertebrae. This requires lift from the shoulders, supported by the action of forearms and the hands.

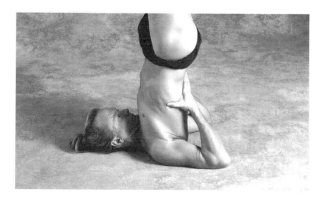

Great care must be taken in both the Shoulderstand and the Headstand that not only the correct foundation support is established but also that the whole of the rest of the body is activated against the force of gravity so as to avoid pressure on the neck.

In seated forward extensions, the foundation is the back of the legs and the bottom of the pelvis. In order to use the legs effectively as supports from which the spine can relax and release itself freely along its whole length, they must make full contact with the floor. This means they must be able to straighten. If our hamstrings are not completely

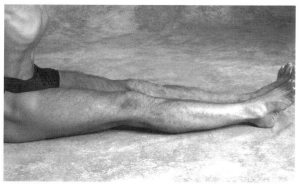

free this will be difficult, and much attention, and judicious effort, must be given to the feet and thighs to bring the backs of the knees down so that the legs are straight and in maximum contact with the floor.

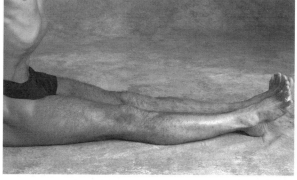

This is made possible by repetitive work in the standing poses.

In some floor postures, such as the various Marichyasana, the foundation is one leg and buttock, and one foot. Here the same principles apply. Both the straight and the bent leg and foot are active, with the weight spread evenly between them, and equally across their individual surfaces.

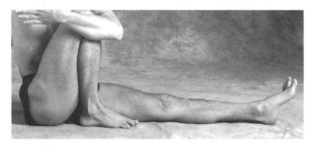

The Limbs

The way that we use our limbs to support the foundation is crucial. The activity of the muscles of the limbs is subtle. The muscles are used not to articulate the bones, as *Asana* is a static process in terms of external movement, but to cradle and support them: to make them stable. This involves lengthening and sealing muscle groups into the bones. This is a use of motor muscles which is unfamiliar to us. Again we must be patient in learning it. It does not involve intense muscular contractions causing shortening in the centre of the muscle body. When this happens the muscles tend to pull away from the bone, destabilizing them as if in preparation to move them.

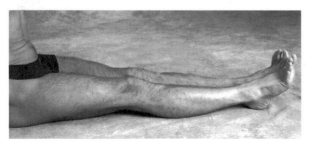

But in *asana* we wish to stabilize and immobilize the bones. So we must learn to contract only the ends of the muscle body, at the origin and insertion, so that this lengthens the centre of the muscle and flattens it in against the bone.

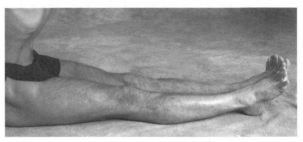

This sealing process also has the complementary, desired effect of opening the joints. It is experienced as a sucking sensation of the muscles into the bone which creates space under the skin, and a feeling of emptiness in the bones. In between these two areas of spaciousness, there is a feeling of energetic solidity that is quite free from strain or tension.

This sealing process also serves the purpose of straightening the legs, by bringing the thighs in line with the calves, while opening and centring the knee joint. This is necessary to stabilize the legs, and allow them to transmit the even stability of the feet through the pelvis to the spine.

If the legs are not straightened, they do not provide the necessary effortless stability to release the spine, the pelvic floor and the core of the body.

Care must be taken to prevent hyperextension of the legs in standing postures.

To prevent this, enough weight must be kept on the ball of the foot, the front thigh must be sealed fully into the bone, and the calf muscle lifted into the bone so that the shinbone moves away from the heel.

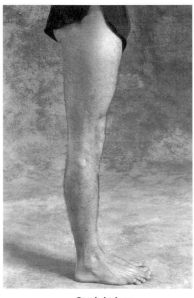

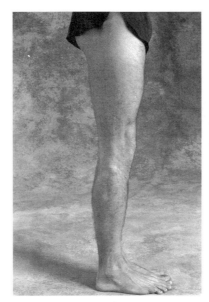

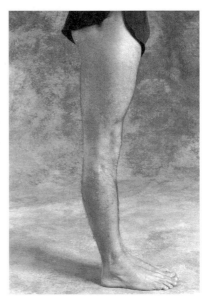

Straight legs **Bent legs** **Hyperextending legs**

33

The same is true when the legs are apart and feet turned. Then weight must be brought to the ball of the front foot, by pushing the weight from the back foot. The legs must both be straight with the front leg thigh pulling the thighbone out of the knee joint, and the front leg calf lifting the shinbone out of the back of the knee joint.

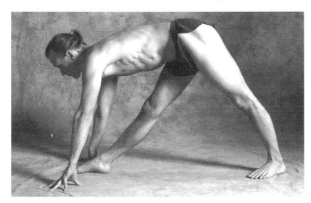

This sealing process is also used in the legs, and the arms also, even when they are not connected to the foundation. For example, by sealing the legs in this way during inversions the legs are lifted, almost squeezed, out of the pelvis, relieving the foundation of some of their weight.

This sealing action of the muscles of the limbs is more than an anatomical process. It is a physiological one also. It promotes a deep release in the tissues, nerves, capillaries, veins, ducts and channels of the skin and joints. This allows a fuller, freer flow of

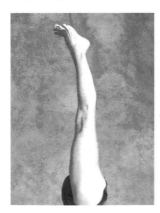

liquids and nerve impulses. This process is also activated in the trunk and spine through the *bandhas*. When the surface and periphery are made stable, the depths and centre can release. This is a basic principle of *asana*, whereby we access the deeper, subtle aspects of our being.

In the arms this action is brought about mainly through the use of the hands. By lengthening into the fingers, and broadening the palms the muscles of the arm are lengthened and sealed.

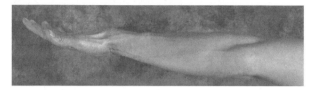

This action is part of the overall manner in which the arms are extended, straightened and stabilized when they are held free in space, whether vertically or horizontally.

This same lengthening and sealing action is used again in Downward Dog pose to support the foundation by transmitting its even stability up into the shoulders and back muscles to release the spine.

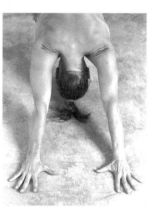

Some people must take care that they do not hyperextend the arm at the elbow joint. If this tends to happen, then they must be consciously shortened until the respective muscles establish their correct lengths.

This action is in fact a spirallic one. As the arm extends out of the shoulder joint, or the wrist in dogpose, the upper arm rotates outwards while the lower arm rotates inwards. This gives the arms the strength and stability of a rope. To get a feel for this extend one arm out of the armpit parallel to the floor. Broaden the palm, lengthen the fingers and turn the palm to face the ceiling.

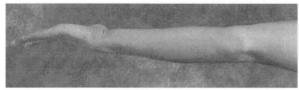

Then without turning the upper arm or the bones of the elbow, turn the palm back to face the floor so that the wrist and forearm turn with it.

This is the spiral.

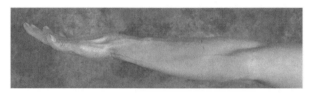

This is especially important in dog pose, and helps to adjust the top spine and chest. The legs also work spirallically in many poses, including dog pose. The backwards action of the inner ankle is balanced by the backwards action of the outer hip. In this way top and bottom of the leg oppose each other and create the energetic stability of a spirallic momentum.

Knees

Padmasana, or Lotus position, is the popularized ideal of *yogasana*. However it utilizes extreme mobility in hips, knees and ankles. A mobility that very few Westerners have. Therefore great care must be taken when attempting not only Lotus, but any bent leg position. This includes half-lotus, and other forward extensions with one leg bent. Of the hips, knees and ankles, the knees are not only the most mobile, but the most vulnerable. Consequently it is the joint that takes the force when we try to impose Lotus, or similar leg bending actions, before we are ready. This readiness is mainly in the hips, and is cultivated mainly in standing postures. Between them the standing postures open up the pelvis to its full capacity and range of movement, making this movement available for more advanced postures.

When attempting *Padmapascimottanasana* in the Preparatory Series, or Lotus variations in yoga classes, take great care. Be patient. Do not force anything. In bending the leg support the knee and the foot, and releasing the flesh of calf and thigh from each other, bring the bones of the shin and thigh as close to each other as possible before moving the foot towards the other thigh. This action is NOT done by pulling the foot towards the thigh. Rather the foot is transported passively on to the thigh by moving its thigh in towards the other one.

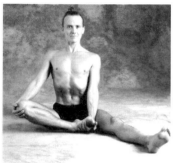

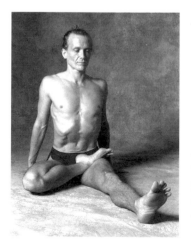

This will utilize the mobility of the hip socket to bring the foot into place. If there is not enough mobility in the hip socket the foot will not comfortably reach the opposite thigh. It must not be forced into position. Doing so will lead to damage to the knee that may be irreparable. Do not cultivate attachment to appearances. You only have two knees, and you need them both. If the foot does not freely reach, then place it under the thigh, so that it makes the same relationship to its hip but without pressure in the knee or ankle.

This is the first leg position for *Sukhapadapascimottanasana*.

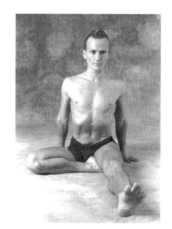

Whenever you might attempt full Lotus, begin in the way described above. Then bring the second leg across in exactly the same manner.

Because the first leg is already up, twisting the second knee is more likely as the leg must be raised higher to get over the first. This can be avoided. Take care. Take just as much care uncrossing the legs. It is here that damage is often done. As you release the top leg take hold of its knee and ankle and, while cupping the kneecap with one hand, use the one on the ankle to rotate the shinbone away from you as you move the leg down. This should avoid pinching in the inner front knee.

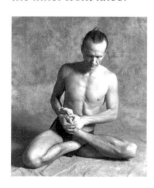
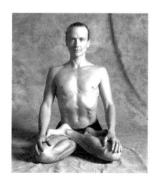

When the front leg is bent in some of the standing poses it must be positioned precisely. The angle between the shin bone and thigh bone should be 90 degrees.

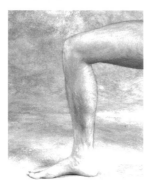 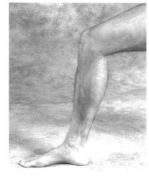

Correct   **Incorrect**

This ensures that the body of the shin bone in its vertical position can provide the maximum resistance to gravity. If this is not so, then the thigh muscles have to overwork to resist gravity and maintain stability. This not only means that the leg becomes tired, but the correct sealing action cannot occur due to excess contraction of the quadriceps. Once you have awakened the intelligence of the feet and legs you can establish this line through the feet. The position of the knee relative to the heel indicates the weight distribution on the feet. If the weight is forward on the foot, the knee comes forward.

If the weight is back on the heel, the knee tends to be behind the heel. If the weight is more on the inner edge of the foot, the knee is falling inwards.

If the weight is more on the outer edge, the knee is falling outwards.

While the knee in front of or behind the heel is tiring, to the left or right it is dangerous. It twists and puts pressure on the knee. This strains the ligaments of the knee, and can lead to tearing. This can happen in everyday life, especially when running on uneven ground, and using the clutch and brake while driving.

36

Hands and Feet

Even when the feet are not part of the foundation they are of great importance. So also the hands. Being at the very periphery of our physical structure, they stand in complementary opposition to its centre: the core of our body. This creates an intense potential dynamic between them, that if activated can charge the whole body with vitality. The hands and feet then are always kept alive, vibrant and active, while the core of the body is kept soft, passive and receptive. The blocked energy of tension in the core of the body is then drawn out to the periphery, and distributed into the whole body as potential for activity, nourishment or rejuvenation.

When the feet are not on the floor, in sitting forward extensions, inversions, etc., they should be alive and energized. This can be difficult to learn, as our feet, locked away all day in restricting shoes, tend to be unresponsive in the beginning. They may either remain inert, or become somewhere tense. At least when they are on the floor, bearing weight, they have something to work against.

The ball of the foot should be broad, and open. It should be further from the ankle than the heel: this keeps the ankle open and helps to lengthen the shinbone out of the knee joint also.

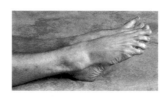

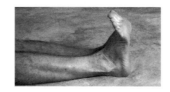

However it should not be pushed blindly forward like a dancer. This cramps the ball of the foot, overstretches the front ankle, tightening the Achilles tendon. All four sides of the ankle joint should be extended evenly. This means that none can reach their limits, but none is blocked either. Neither must the feet be pulled back, overstretching the Achilles, blocking the front

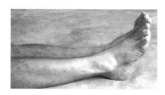

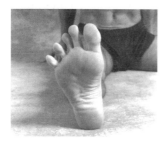

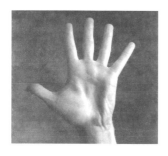

ankle and shortening the shin bone.

There should be length also between the inner ankle and the inner heel. The toes should be extending gently out of the ball of the foot, upwards rather than forwards without being tense or tightening their tendons.

The furthest point from the navel and ankle should be the centre of the ball of the foot, not the ball of the big toe, nor the toes.

When standing, the ankle is the joint closest to the floor. It bears the whole weight of the body and is often restricted. We must learn to open the ankle joint evenly and fully, so that it sits centred and freely in between the foot and the leg. When standing, if weight tends to roll to the outer edge of the foot, hit the inner ankle bone back hard, and continuously. This will help to maintain the activity of the inner plane of the legs while keeping them straight.

The quality of the hands while they are held in space is similar to that when supporting Downward Dog pose. The palms are kept broad and long, this creates arching between the heel and the base of the fingers, the fingers long, the sides of the wrists extended evenly.

The charged quality of the hands and feet not only draws energy outwards from the centre, but also acts as a seal to reverse it back in again towards the centre.

The Pelvis

The pelvis is the fulcrum between the legs and the trunk. The activity of the feet and legs cannot reach and support the spine if it is lost in the pelvis. Therefore the pelvis must be open and aligned in order to transmit the stability and support of the lower body to the spine. When the body is inverted, this remains true in the opposite direction.

However most of us carry tension throughout the musculature of the pelvis: in the pelvic floor; in the hip joints; in the sacroiliac joint; in the pubic abdomen. This tension restricts our use of the legs, and movement of the spine. For the pelvis is the soil in which the spine is rooted, via the sacrum and the coccyx. This tension is effectively released through continuous practice of the full range of standing poses. They will systematically and progressively release the full mobility of the pelvis. Without complete freedom in the pelvis, complete release and balanced lengthening of the spinal column is not possible.

One of the main problems people encounter, however, is that due to weakness in the abdomen, and lower back problems, the whole pelvis is tilted.

The top front comes forward and down, the bottom back comes backward and up. This is the classic swayback position. This can initially be addressed from the position of the hip bones.

Simply lifting the hip bones up and away from the thighs will begin to compensate for this distortion.

As you do this you should feel the groins opening, stretching and lengthening; the front of your body will feel longer. This does not involve tilting the top of the pelvis backwards nor the bottom forwards.

This movement **must** be initiated from the hipbones at the front, and **not** from the coccyx at the back. If you do it from behind, the tailbone tuck, although the hipbones will lift the sacroiliac joints will tighten, the thigh bones will be pushed forwards, and the pelvis becomes insensitive and dull, breaking the continuity between legs and spine.

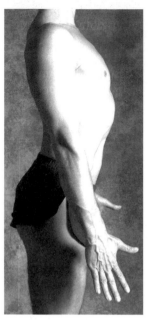

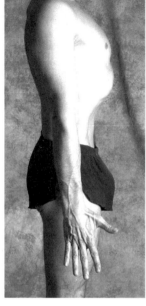

Swayback

38

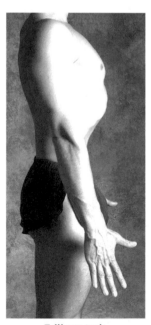

Tailbone tuck

Another related problem is displacement of the sacrum itself. One or more edges of the sacrum is not embedded truly in the pelvis. This is compensated for, and prevented, by drawing the sacrum inwards and upwards. This should be done evenly, left-right and top-bottom. It should not resemble the tailbone tuck, nor tilt the bottom of the pelvis forward, nor the top backwards. This adjustment is subtle, but vital. By engaging the bottom of the spine fully into the pelvic support, the lower back is relieved of taking any undue strain. This is especially important in backward bending poses, and requires the support of the legs. It is achieved from the front, not the back. The deep lateral muscles of the pubic abdomen engage, flattening the lower abdomen and drawing the sacrum in. It is in fact one of the effects of a judicious *Mulabandha*.

Because of these problems, and others, the pelvis is often misaligned in Downward Dog pose. This deprives it of its ability to fully rest and rejuvenate. It also prevents the balanced awakening of somatic intelligence for which this pose is especially fruitful. For people with flexible lumbar spines (lower backs), the buttock bones are often pulled too far upwards.

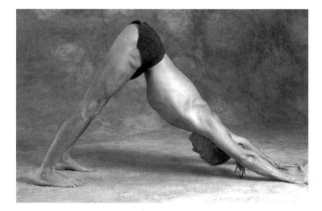

This puts pressure on the lumbar vertebrae and distorts the legs. Others go to the other extreme, imitating the tailbone tuck.

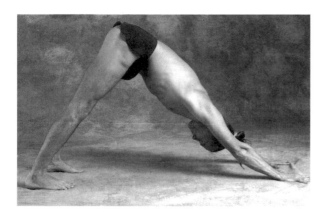

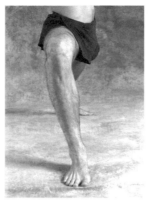

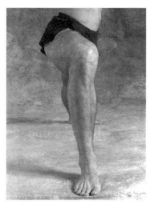

This can also strain the lower back, and deadens the pose. Instead the pelvis should be balanced, with a feeling of ease in the lower back, freedom in the hip sockets, and an overall feeling of vibrant emptiness in the pelvis.

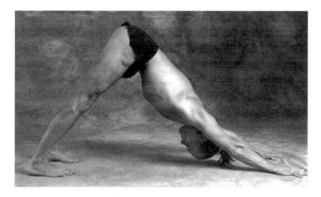

Another common problem is in standing poses such as *Parsvavirabhadrasana*, *Parsvakonasana* variations, and *Utthita Trikonasana*. In these poses only too often the front buttock moves out to the side, away from the opposite groin. This is often accompanied by a leaning of the front knee inwards (see section above on Knees).

The front buttock bone should be kept in line with the knee on the plane of the feet, with the buttock flesh being taken in towards the pubis and back towards the back groin spirallically.

This adjustment needs to be complemented by the action of the front of the back leg thigh: it should press hard straight back in towards the bone and the hamstring. Without this opposing force, the adjustment of tucking the front buttock in can disturb the line of the pelvis. It should also be complemented by the adjustment explained below.

Of the main group of asymmetrical standing poses, in which the legs are used differently from each other, there are two kinds in terms of the alignment of the pelvis: those in which the pelvis is aligned along the axis described by the feet, and those in which it bisects that plane. In both cases the true line requires effort. In the case of those, such as *Utthita Trikonasana*, *Parsvakonasana* and *Parsvavirabhadrasana*, which occur on a single plane, the tendency is for the back hip to roll forwards off the plane of the legs.

39

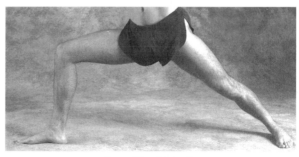

Leg rolling forwards

It must be kept rolled back. It is supported in this by hitting the outer edge of the back knee backwards, so that the whole of the back leg is spiralling away from the front one. This requires that the back leg be kept straight so it can absorb and transmit the turn. This requires the support, through resistance to this action, of the ankle and foot.

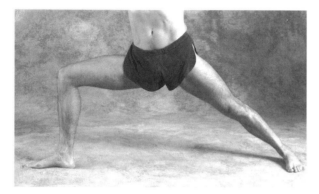

Hip rolled back

40

In the case of those postures in which the pelvis dissects the plane of the legs (*Parvritatrikonasana, Parsvottanasana, Virabhadrasana*), the difficulty is of bringing the back hip into line with the front. This depends upon flexibility in the hip sockets. It is supported by turning the back leg groin back, while hitting its inner knee backwards so that the whole leg is turning back from the inside and the outside of the leg turns forward, bringing the hip into line. This also requires that the back leg be kept straight so it can absorb and transmit the turn.

Abdomen

The quality of the abdomen is a vital feature of Hatha Yoga. Misuse of the abdomen can lead to weakening of the lower back, inhibited breathing, hypertension and insensitivity. It should neither be hard nor soft; neither tense nor dormant. It should be long, hollow, passive, firm and stable. In this state it acts as a firm support for the lumbar spine,

the diaphragm, and the activity of the ribcage. With only a very few exceptions, this holds true for all *Asana* regardless of the external shape. In some cases this is easier than others. Even in many poses where this seems extremely difficult (*Navasana, Sarvangasana*) it should be attempted. In some however, it should not, mainly those where the spine is intentionally rounded, with the top front spine drawn towards the bottom front (*Ardhapindasana, Karnapidasana*).

The abdomen is soft when the muscles are short and inactive. Often this shows as bulging around and below the navel.

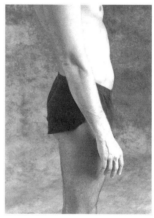

The abdomen is hard when the muscles are contracted. This tends to pull the bottom of the breastbone down, collapsing the collarbones and restricting the ribcage.

To lengthen the abdomen, the muscles in the abdominal wall must first be passive. Then we lift the ribcage away from the pelvis evenly. The armpits should lift away from the hipbones, but the shoulders should not lift towards the ears, but remain relaxed.

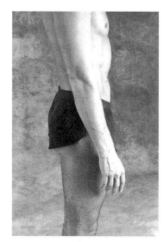

The main quality of the abdomen is that it should be hollow. This means the abdominal wall does not stick out, but draws in towards the spine. This is not

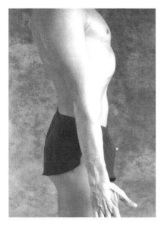

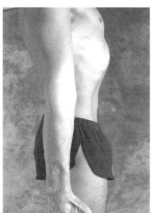

done by pushing the abdominal wall back, but by lifting and broadening the ribcrest, and sucking the solar plexus in from above. Although the abdomen does become firm, this is due to its lifting up and in. As the muscles lengthen they increase their tonal quality. The vertical muscle body is not contracting, however.

For further details on the use of the abdomen, refer to the section on the *bandhas* explaining the action of *Uddiyanabandha* (page 49).

Chest

The chest, or ribcage, is the seat of the lungs. It needs to be given the maximum possibility of opening. Only then can the lungs breathe freely and fully. The quality of the ribcage should complement that of the abdomen. It should be broad, active and full, the abdomen long, passive and empty. When lifting the ribcage away from the pelvis, thereby lengthening both the abdomen and the spine, the chest should broaden. This broadening begins at the ribcrest, where it is easier, and ends at the collarbones, where it is harder. While broadening the ribcrests they should not be thrust forward, nor should the bottom of the breastbone jut forwards.

Rather, the ribcrests should almost tuck inwards, so that the floating ribs feel as if they are drawing towards the hipbones. At the same time the skin under the floating ribs should seal in against the liver and the stomach.

Of course, in some positions (*Ardhapindasana*, *Karnapidasana*), the chest cannot maintain these qualities. Then concentrate on opening and broadening the back of the ribcage, allowing the back lungs to open more.

The way that we use the ribcage as a whole is connected to the use of the breastbone. Care must be taken that, in attempting to open the chest, the bottom breastbone is not pushed forward: rather it should slightly tuck down and in. The top breastbone should lift up and slightly out.

The position of the shoulder blades is also important. They should be drawn in to the body and down, keeping breadth between them, stimulating the lungs to open and supporting the thoracic vertebrae. The collarbones should normally be kept parallel to the pubic bones, so that the trunk and spine are not tilting to one side. This is especially prone to occur in sitting spinal twists.

Neck

The neck is a very vulnerable part of our body. Besides which it has to carry not only the heavy weight of the head, but the even heavier weight of our incessant thoughts. Great care must be taken when moving it. It should never be jerked, pulled or pushed. Move slowly, smoothly and with due sensitivity.

When the head is fully or partially up, the back neck shortens. Care must be taken to keep as much space between the back of the vertebrae as possible. If not they will jam, the muscles will tighten, with pain and restricted movement soon to follow. The key to this is lifting the chin forwards and the base of the skull upwards as you take your head back.

41

When the head is taken down to the chest, care must be taken that the back of the neck is soft first. Also that the movement is one of relaxing the back of the neck as the head goes down, not one of pulling down. Neck muscles are often tight, and will not freely allow the full downwards movement of the chin. In this case we have to wait patiently for the back neck muscles to soften and lengthen. This can be assisted by the Shoulderstand and variations, provided they are not overdone.

The standing poses can also help the neck, as a result of the turning of the head to the left and right, as can twists. When this is done the vertebrae of the cervical spine (in the neck) must be rotated on their axis. This axis should be a direct continuation of the thoracic (upper) spine. The neck is part of the spine. When turning the head to left and right, in standing poses and other postures such as sitting twists, it must be treated as such. While the neck can turn much more than the thoracic spine, it should turn along the same axis. Otherwise the sides of the neck will distort: one too short, one too long.

In both Headstand and variations, and Shoulderstand and its cycle, weight is carried by the neck. Care must be taken to ensure that the neck is adequately supported in this. This is done by lifting each part of the body against gravity so the load on the neck is less, and by ensuring that the body's weight is spread across the rest of the foundation provided by arms and hands. Care must also be taken to position the head and neck symmetrically, so that the muscles on each side are worked evenly and do not become distorted.

Spine

Judicious attention to the position, shape and quality of the pelvis, abdomen, chest and neck will of course determine the shape and quality of the spine. While we often use the adjective 'straight' to qualify the noun 'spine', this is a distortion. The spine is not and must not be straight. Rather it

should be fully extended or elevated, with space, and therefore freedom of movement, between each of the vertebrae. This will express its natural curves. The key to this is the use of the *bandhas*. When we are able to perform *Mulabandha* fully, the sacrum is brought in line. This releases the lower back and the lumbar vertebrae. When we are able to perform *Uddiyanabandha* fully, the lumbar spine and thoracic spine lengthen, the lumbar vertebrae move back and out, the thoracic vertebrae lift inwards and upwards. This compensates for the

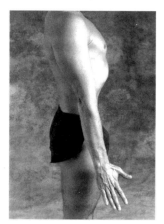

common lumbar and thoracic distortions, and brings the spine into its natural line, with two gentle, opposing curves at the lumbar and thoracic spine complemented by two lesser opposing and complementary curves at the sacrum and the neck.

Of course, the spine can be lifted and lengthened without direct use of the *bandhas*. Then we have to create space between the armpits and hipbones, between the ribcrests and pubis; we have to adjust the shape and position of the floating ribs, fixed ribs and breastbone; we have to align the collarbones, the shoulders and the shoulder blades; we have to adjust the hipbones, the sacrum, the buttocks and perineum. All of these things, however, occur simultaneously as a result of the *bandhas*. Initially the nerves and muscles are unable to fully activate the *bandhas*, but with constant repetition they can, and do.

An unsupported spine will not show the four natural curves. Most commonly the tailbone will stick out, the lumbar will arch forward, the thoracic spine and neck will collapse. It takes time to

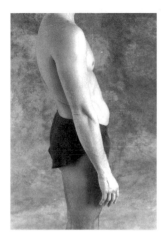

change this. All of the muscles of the body are involved, not just those of the trunk, and must be re-educated and developed in harmony with each other.

The Basic Principles of Alignment

The easy stability that is alignment encompasses structural integrity (earth), functional freedom (water), energetic harmony (fire), internal spaciousness (air) and effortless attention (space). This is *Asana*. This state is supported and indicated by a number of qualities or principles. Enumerating these principles is somewhat arbitrary and personal. Do not get caught in one at the expense of another. Nor see them as separate from each other or the whole that they point towards, or even see them as the whole that they simply reflect.

1 **Opposition** This comes from balancing any applied line of force with equal and opposing ones, in a spirallic momentum, that take into account the following poles:

> left/right
> top/bottom
> front/back
> inside/outside
> centre/periphery.

2 **Stability** This comes from a combination of sealing the muscles of the body into the bone, by lengthening them, and opposition.

3 **Balance** This comes from an even and integrated distribution of action and awareness across those same poles:

> left/right
> top/bottom
> front/back
> inside/outside
> centre/periphery.

4 **Effortlessness** This comes from the release that stabilizing and balancing the outer body through opposition gives to the core of the body, the body as a whole and each individual part of the body.

5 **Emptiness** This comes from the effortless balancing of stable lines of opposing force across the five poles of each part of the body and throughout the whole of the body.

43

6

VINYASA: THE QUALITY OF MOVEMENT

Vinyasa has so many different applications that many of them are often overlooked in the practice of Hatha Yoga. *Vinyasa* implies continuity, fluidity, connectivity, setting out and returning to the same place, step-by-step progression. In all cases the key, which makes the process *vinyasa*, is the synchronization of movement and breath. While in any given application the process of *vinyasa* is simple, its overall implications are extremely sophisticated and far-reaching.

The Vinyasa

In *Asana* practice continuity simply means that we do not break the flow of awareness, internalization, concentration or action in between postures. To maintain this flow we use the rhythm of our breathing to guide us out of one posture, and into the next. Very often this is by way of another group of postures, often known as The Vinyasa. These postures are designed as counterbalance to the posture before, and preparation for the posture after. There are a number of varieties of this in the Vinyasa section of Part III.

Here, *vinyasa* has a very important function. It is not just a question of muscular compensation and preparation. It ensures that whatever opening of the body occurred in the previous *Asana* is assimilated into the body as a whole as a potentiality, rather than a fixed movement. It also gives us a chance to re-establish the free rhythm of our breathing if that has been disturbed by the challenge of the posture. By re-establishing movement it gives us a break from the stillness of *Asana*, which itself can be deeply challenging. It also allows for a recentring of the body's nervous and energy systems, and of the mind.

Synchronization

The key to this simple but potent process is the breathing. Each movement in the *vinyasa* sequence is synchronized exactly with either the inhalation or the exhalation. This synchronization must be exact if it is to deliver its full potential. There should be continuous movement of both body and breath, with no resting or pausing for breath or body to catch up with the other. The movement is initiated exactly with its inhalation or exhalation, and finishes exactly when that phase of the breath ends. Exactly. The rhythm of body movement mirrors exactly that of the breath. The speed of body movement is determined by the rate of breathing. The more slowly you are breathing, the more slowly you move.

Of course this also means that the shorter the range of movement, the slower you must move. This is because the breath has primacy in this relationship. Never hurry the breath. The body must adjust its speed of movement to that of the breath. Not the other way round. Making the breath follow the body movement stimulates the sympathetic nervous activity: hardens the muscles, shortens and speeds up the breath, increases heart beat, speeds up brain activity, drains the internal organs of blood, overstimulates the glands. Whereas adjusting the body movement to fit the rhythm of the breath stimulates the parasympathetic nervous activity: softens the muscles, deepens and slows down the breath, slows down the heart beat, slows down the brain, engorges the internal organs with blood, and balances the glands.

Exact synchronization of body and breath also has a profound effect on the mind. By harmonizing the anatomical, voluntary muscles and nerves with the physiological, involuntary muscles and nerves, it draws the mind deeper. It elicits a profound stillness and quietness as attention's energy is drawn away from the stimuli which invade the sensory motor nervous system, and is brought to bear upon the internal environment of the autonomic nervous system. Besides which the absolute concentration required of feeling and adjusting the rate of movement of the anatomical muscles, so that they synchronize exactly with the respiratory muscles, brings the mind to a very deep, clear, stable focus. This effect can be felt immediately by anyone. It does not depend on strength, flexibility, stamina or structural freedom. It clarifies, again, the supremacy of the breath over movement, of quality over quantity.

This principle of breath-determined movement between postures finds subtle application with regard to the exact manner of entering and leaving a posture. The coming and going of a posture are not separate from it. Their quality will affect that of the posture. This again means that the steps that we take to enter and leave a posture are synchronized with our breathing. This means that we can enter a posture, and leave it, slowly, safely and smoothly. This smoothness is part of the continuity aspect of *vinyasa*. It soothes, tranquillizes and harmonizes the mind. Its presence is the source of grace in *Asana*.

Entering a posture involves clearly delineable movements or steps. Each one of those steps is synchronized with either an inhalation or an exhalation. The principle for determining which to use is simple enough. If the movement opens the front of the body, inhale. If it closes the front of the body, exhale. This principle helps you to determine which actions constitute a movement. A movement is a group of actions, or even a single action, that brings you further into, or out of, the pose, on the breath. To leave a posture we apply the same principle of breath-determined steps.

In the Postures section (Part III), instruction is given as to how to breathe and move together when entering and leaving a posture. From these instructions you will grasp the principle involved. As your body opens up and your mind becomes more focused, you will be able to group more actions together into a single movement. You must still adhere to the breath/body synchronization principle, making sure that anatomical movement supports and is supported by physiological movement.

The exact manner of entering any pose is not fixed, nor is it arbitrary. It always involves synchronizing the body's movements with the breath. And it always involves conscious use of the breath and body to penetrate a pose. Usually this takes a number of gradual steps. As somatic intelligence awakens, the number of steps (breath-related groups of movements) can be reduced. Eventually the pose can be entered in a single step, on either an inhalation or an exhalation. The steps taken are determined by the capacity and limitations of your body at any given time, which are not always the same. This step-by-step progression into a posture ensures that we do not exceed our limits by imposing an unreachable goal on ourselves. It is a specific, subtle application of the principle of *vinyasa krama*.

Vinyasa Krama

Vinyasa krama is the technique of progressing step by step from the known to the unknown. This means constructing a practice sequence, or establishing a posture, from clearly defined blocks, or steps. *Vinyasa krama* underlies the order of postures in a practice format. This is at the heart of Vinniyoga practice. It is based on an understanding of the progressive and balancing effects of the various postures. It also underlies the manner of entering and leaving a posture.

As our bodies become more open, less restricted, we can exercise greater freedom in our choice and sequencing of postures. When our bodies are free from habitual tension we can sequence postures more according to their energetic and psychological effects. But until then we must respect the actual, albeit restricted, capacity of our body. Therefore, where the traditional practice formats present a challenge to our bodies which can put them at risk, they must be adapted according to safe, effective structural principles. The esoteric knowledge required to guide us in sequencing for energetic enhancement is beyond all but the most dedicated and experienced practitioners.

The traditional sequencing formats of Hatha Yoga begin with the dynamic Sun Salutations. In physical terms, this warms up the body: softening muscles, opening joints. Then follows a series of standing poses. These gently awaken cellular intelligence, the legs, pelvis and spine, without asking the spine to make any extreme movements. Once mobilized the spine can be stretched forwards, backwards or to the side in twists. Of these three movements, forward bends are the easiest and most familiar, backbends the most difficult and intense. The spine is warmed up further, and mobility of the pelvis developed, with forward extensions. Twists are then utilized as preparations for stronger movements of the spine, both in intense forward bends and backbends. When fully warmed up it is exposed to backbends.

Within this basic structure – Sun Salutation, standing poses, forward bends, twists, backbends – many variations are possible. These variations embrace different degrees of flexibility in all the different muscles and joints. Different bodies prosper with different sequences, depending upon their personal limitations and capabilities. However these sequences must respect the natural laws of physical movement. This means that joints must be opened gradually so as not to strain them. Postures that work more deeply into the muscles and joints should follow those that are more superficial.

Simpler postures should be used to rest after more demanding ones. It is simply a matter of common sense combined with sensitivity and anatomical awareness.

Some Hatha Yoga postures require extreme joint mobility beyond that of most Westerners. This capacity must be cultivated patiently and gently. To overlook the structural limitations of the body and requirements of a posture, in order to access the energetic process is putting the cart before the horse. If we spend a little time dealing with the realities of our structural limitations, we will find ourselves able to drink more deeply of the energetic effects of the traditional postures and formats. When the time comes, when the body is free of tension, then the energetic effects of Hatha Yoga become available and apparent.

Until then the body must be awakened and opened patiently and systematically. This fact underlies the posture sequencing of the Dynamic Yoga Series. They allow you to cultivate a gradual, stable opening of the skeleto/muscular systems while at the same time awakening the body's cellular intelligence. They are directly based on the *yoga chikitsa* sequencing, used not only in Ashtanga Vinyasa Yoga, but also in its derivative forms. The practice of *yoga chikitsa* not only restructures the body. It also endows us with a deep practical understanding of the body, its capacity and its intelligence. The *yoga chikitsa* postures are like letters or words sequenced for a particular purpose: freeing the physical structure from restriction. When this has been achieved, these words are free for us to make our own poetry with.

Heat

One of the most obvious effects of continuity is to gradually build up physical heat. This heat affects the whole of the inside of the body. As the body warms up muscles soften, ligaments loosen, joints open and excess liquid is driven to the surface. We start to sweat. The sweat has two functions. First it acts as a medium to transport toxins to the surface where they can be discharged. This is similar to the fever process of burning out toxins. Secondly it acts as insulation. The sweat acts like a wet suit. It coats the body with a thermal layer that then keeps inside the heat being generated. Then this heat can be utilized and transformed by the *bandhas*. If the sweat we create is continually dripping off our bodies, we have to use up more heat to replace it. This uses up excessive energy, and exhausts us. We should not therefore wipe sweat away from our body, not even from the face. Therefore we must pay attention to how much we are sweating, and make sure that our activity is not producing a drain on our energy through loss of physical heat. If the sweat is dripping off us, we should slow down a little, and return to a concern for quality rather than quantity. The heat that we require of Hatha Yoga is subtle internal, transforming heat. Not gross, external, draining heat.

Vinyasa, then, is a fundamental aspect of *Asana*. It gives our practice grace and effortlessness, safety and power. Without it our practice is greatly diminished.

47

7

THE BANDHAS: THE QUALITY OF ENERGY

The *Bandhas* are at the very core of Hatha Yoga practice. They represent the most subtle and potent difference between the postures of Hatha Yoga and gymnastic exercises. Through them we deeply internalize our awareness, generate, contain and transform heat and energy, and transform the activity of our nervous system. This influences both our mind and our body. The *bandhas* are often called the spiritual doorway, through which we enter a dimension of ourselves and reality not often reached naturally.

The *bandhas* involve muscular adjustments related more to our physiological than anatomical bodies, more to our involuntary muscles than our voluntary muscles. Therefore they are initially very elusive, but with practice become quite natural. Deliberately engaging these muscles during *Asana* has a profound effect not only on our muscular body. It also effects our skeleton and the central nervous system. By engaging the sacrum, lumbar, thoracic and cervical vertebrae, the spine is aligned, its central channel opened. By stimulating the solar plexus energy is generated and transformed. By stimulating the perineal body and the sacral ganglia the peripheral and sympathetic nervous systems are quietened, the parasympathetic nervous system activated and the central nervous system is charged with energy. This can be felt clearly in the spine, but also in the brain.

Jalandharabandha

Jalandharabandha involves lowering the chin on to the breastbone, so as to change the shape and size of the throat.

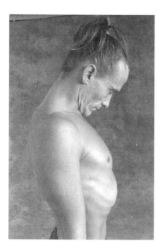

This slows the breathing down, making it more audible. However the chin is not in contact with breastbone in all *Asana* except Shoulderstand variations.

To bring about the energetic effect of *Jalandharabandha* without its overt anatomical aspect, one has to adjust the throat internally. This is done by shaping the throat as if you were about to pronounce a hard 'c' or 'g', but without doing so. This elicits contact between throat and palate which causes an energetic seal while slowing down the breath and making it audible. This contact allows you to suck the inhalation in from deep in the lungs, and to resist the exhalation from the level of the palate.

The sound resulting from *Jalandharabandha* is the distinguishing characteristic of *Ujjayi* breathing. It should be a soft, smooth, rhythmic, potent sound. It should not be harsh, forced or imposed. It happens naturally due to the shape of the throat and the quality of the breath.

Uddiyanabandha

Uddiyanabandha involves sucking the solar plexus in and up.

When practised in isolation this is done when the lungs are empty, and occurs as a result of a pressure differential caused by lifting the ribcage as if inhaling without drawing air in. The pressure differential caused by not inhaling draws the abdominal wall and organs up and in. However, because the normal rhythm of breathing is maintained during *Asana*, a modified, partial version of *Uddiyana* must then be used.

To bring about the energetic and anatomical effects of *Uddiyanabandha* while breathing requires that the respiratory muscles of inhalation act in unison with the transverse muscles of the pubic abdomen to stabilize and lengthen the abdomen, stabilize and lift the lungs, and thereby draw the abdominal wall and organs up and in.

49

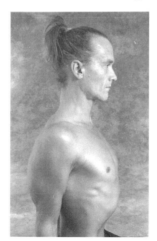 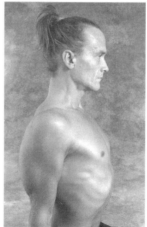

Uddiyanabandha, lungs empty Uddiyanabandha, lungs full

From these illustrations both the difference and similarities can be seen between *Uddiyana* with lungs empty and full. Muscles usually used only during inhalation are consciously kept active during exhalation to create the effect of *Uddiyanabandha*. Rather than inhibiting the exhalation this challenges, refines and focuses it.

The abdomen is not tightened or shortened, nor is it pushed back against the spine.

Uddiyanabandha is a vertical momentum, lengthening the abdomen and spine. It is initiated from the ribcage, by lifting it while broadening it. This lift is initiated at the back sides and top, rather than the front. The broadening begins at the ribcrest and rises to the collarbones. It elicits a deep suction on the solar plexus, which also draws the abdominal organs up and in.

Uddiyana polarizes the chest and abdomen, enhancing the charge in each and between them. The chest is full, active and broad. The abdomen is empty, passive and long.

The more deeply you can clarify this polarity the more effective will be *Uddiyana*.

EXPLORING UDDIYANABANDHA

To develop a sense of *Uddiyana* during respiration, place the legs in *Baddhakonasana* (page 180) or *Virasana* (page 234), and then lie back on a bolster or, if your back permits, the floor. Entering the pose, feel the lengthening of the abdomen and broadening of the ribcage that it elicits. Adjust the muscles in your trunk to enhance both the length of the abdomen and breadth of the ribcage. Increase the distance between the pubic bone and the breastbone to the maximum. Broaden the ribcrests to the maximum as you inhale. As you inhale, resist puffing out the abdomen. Rather, take the air high and broad into the chest, front, sides and back. The upper abdomen should never rise higher than the top of the ribcrests. Instead as you inhale it should open by broadening along with the ribcrests. Keep this as your focus while both

inhaling and exhaling. Keep the abdominal wall passive, with no muscular contractions.

Mulabandha

Mulabandha involves sucking the perineal body and pelvic floor upwards. This is initiated by a flattening of the pubic abdomen, which draws the sacrum in. The pubic abdomen covers that part of the abdomen that goes down within the pelvis. It begins at the pubis, widening out to the hipbones. This flattening is initiated at the edges of the pubic abdomen, in the groins below the hip bones.

A deep *Uddiyana* will automatically elicit *Mulabandha*. In isolation *Mulabandha* is activated in the pubic abdomen. It then affects the sacrum and the pelvic floor, by drawing both inwards and upwards. Without tightening the vertical muscles of the abdomen, nor tightening around the navel, the edges of the pubic abdomen near the groins and below the hipbones are engaged, so that the pubic abdomen flattens. Compare these two illustrations:

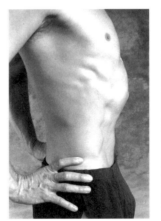 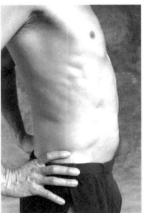

Mulabandha   **Bulging lower abdomen**

The pubic abdomen does not protrude beyond the plane between the hipbones. Nor is it pushed back with a contraction. Neither the navel nor the anus should harden. If you feel with your fingertips you should feel a slight lifting and toning of the side pubic abdomen near the groins, with nothing changing in the centre. If the centre of the pubic abdomen hardens and lifts, try again. A judicious *Mulabandha* produces a softening in the brain and deep in the spine. Any tightening felt in the brain, temples or face indicates error.

EXPLORING MULABANDHA

To develop *Mulabandha* place the legs in *Baddhakonasana* (page 180) or *Virasana* (page 234), and then lie back on a bolster or, if your back permits, the floor. This will naturally stretch and tone the abdominal wall without any voluntary contraction of the muscles. Alternatively go into *Ardhapindasana* (page 212) or *Balasana* (page 226). Focus your attention on the interior of the pelvis. Allow your awareness to saturate this area, absorbing all possible sensations. As you do so, try to discriminate between the pelvic floor and the muscles above inside the pelvic cavity. Be aware of the pelvic floor at the front adjoining the pubic bone. Be aware of the pelvic floor at the back adjoining the coccyx.

The following exercises should be practised in sequence, with a short rest between each. Practise as often as possible, any time, any place, even standing or walking.

1   AWAKENING THE PELVIC FLOOR. Breathing freely, gently but fully, contract and immediately but not hurriedly release all of the muscles of the pelvic floor. Maintain a rhythm of contraction and release that does not involve the higher muscles of the pelvic cavity.
2   ASWINI MUDRA. Breathing freely, gently but fully contract and immediately but not hurriedly release only the anal muscles towards the back of the pelvic floor. Maintain a rhythm of contraction and release that does not involve the higher muscles of the pelvis, nor the muscles near the pubic bone, the urogenital muscles. The muscles you should be using are the muscles you use to prevent defecation.
3   VAJROLI MUDRA. Breathing freely, gently but fully, contract and immediately but not hurriedly release only the urogenital muscles at the front of the pelvic floor. Maintain a rhythm of contraction and release that does not involve the higher muscles of the pelvis, nor the muscles near the coccyx, the anal muscles. The muscles you should be using are the muscles you use to prevent urination.
4   MULABANDHA. Gently flattening the pubic abdomen, feel that while the anal muscles remain passive, the anal mouth narrows as it is drawn in and up. All of the pelvic floor muscles remain passive, yet as it is being acted on it moves and changes shape. Feel the sacrum embed itself more deeply and evenly into the pelvis. *Mulabandha* can be stronger on one side than the other. Try to feel if this is so, and compensate in the way you use the pubic abdominal muscles.

These exercises will all help you to develop the sensitivity and control *Mulabandha* requires. The two classical *mudras* and *Mulabandha* have very different effects, especially on the central nervous system and the quality and orientation of your awareness. Explore.

Each of the *bandhas* can easily be misapplied: *Jalandhara* by tightening the throat and facial muscles and bringing tension into the brain and the core of the body; *Uddiyana* by tightening the muscles of the abdominal wall, especially around the navel, bringing tension to the core of the body and the abdominal organs; and *Mula* by tightening the muscles of the pelvic floor, especially the anal muscles, bringing tension to the core of the body and the lower organs. These restrictive tightenings must be avoided. They disturb the core of the body, overstimulate the sympathetic branch of the peripheral nervous system and displace the central nervous system, externalizing energy and awareness. The combined effect of the *bandhas* is to quieten the peripheral nervous system, access the central nervous system and soften and release the core of the body, internalizing energy and awareness.

To be sure that the *bandhas* are not being done incorrectly, constant awareness of the core of the body must be maintained. The core of the body should remain passive and soft, free from all hardness and tension, at all times. If this quality is disturbed we reduce *Asana* to sophisticated stretch exercise. Therefore you must constantly check the quality of the pelvic floor, abdomen and face, especially ensuring that the anus, navel, eyes and ears are soft. The jaw should remain relaxed while the lips remain closed.

In order to correctly apply the combined grip of *Mulabandha* and *Uddiyanabandha*, a clear understanding of the abdomen is necessary. There should be no tension in the abdomen. The pubic abdomen is active, however. It involves a gentle flattening towards the spine of the inner abdominal wall between the groins. The long vertical muscles of the abdomen must remain passive, so that the central and upper abdomen can be sucked inwards as well as upwards.

The three *bandhas* constitute a single energetic continuum. *Jala* means net, *adhara* means support, *bandha* means seal or lock. Its purpose is to separate the cranial cavity of the skull from the trunk. This is done to prevent the flow of upward moving energy from entering and overstimulating the brain, by keeping it sealed in the trunk. There it can be utilized by *Uddiyanabandha*. *Ud* means upwards, *yana* means flying. It is designed to generate energy and heat, direct energy upwards, and transform physical to subtle energy. Once this subtle energy with its vertical momentum is available it is utilized by *Mulabandha*. *Mula* means root. It refers to the area at the base of the spine, its root. It prevents downwards movement of energy,

and directs the flow of upwards energy into the subtle body.

The circuit of the *bandhas* is one in which energy, initially in the form of heat, is generated and transformed in the centre of the trunk, while the trunk is sealed at the top and bottom to contain and intensify this energy. This creates a spirallic momentum in the trunk of the body, with an upwards inner flow, and a downwards outer flow. The deep upwards momentum of the body's core is supported and complemented by a subtle downwards momentum on the surface. This is felt as the skin of the ribcrests tucking in and sealing the liver and stomach. At the same time the skin on the back moves down, sealing the shoulder blades in. The external energy redirected downwards by the chin lock, is transformed at the solar plexus, and drawn to the pelvis. Energy is then passed upwards into the subtle body through the root lock: *Mulabandha*. This energetic process is one that can be directly experienced with the sensitivity and subtlety that practice brings.

More immediately, however, the *bandhas* have an important impact on posture and breathing. *Mulabandha* engages the sacrum. *Mulabandha* and *Uddiyanabandha* align the lumbar spine. *Uddiyanabandha* engages the thoracic spine and the ribcage. *Jalandhara* engages the thoracic and cervical spine. *Mulabandha* and *Uddiyanabandha* constitute the core adjustment to the body in the form of supporting, releasing, lengthening and aligning the spinal column. This in turn opens the thoracic cavity so that the lungs can move freely and fully, enhancing and releasing our breathing. All of the other physical adjustments support and reflect this one.

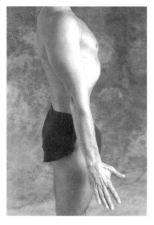 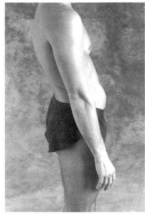

Extended spine   **Unsupported spine**

This fact reflects the universal principle of opposing complementarity overlooked by the dualistic operation of the linear rational mind. Accordingly, energetic and structural processes of the core of the body are reflected at its periphery and surface: i.e. in the limbs, hands and feet. The way that we adjust all of these echoes the action of the *bandhas*, and supports them.

If we examine the action of the legs and arms in standing poses, we find that we engage their full power, giving them maximum stability, by creating a spirallic momentum. This is done by opposing the top of the limbs to the bottom, one turning in each direction. This is rather like twisting the fibres of a rope to give them strength. In the case of the arms this process both lengthens and stabilizes them very simply. To feel this, extend one arm as far out of the shoulder as you can, palm up.

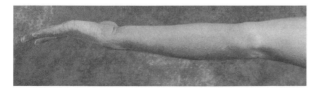

Feel the upwards rotation of the inner front shoulder, and the broadening of the pectoral muscle and chest. Maintaining those qualities in shoulder and chest, carefully turn the wrist so the palm faces down, without turning the upper arm down.

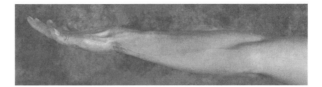

Now the arm is not only longer and stronger but highly energized, with opposition at the elbow. Its quality mirrors that of the trunk, fully charged by the *bandhas*.

Similar spirallic momentums can be felt in the legs. In dog pose, for example, to keep the knees and legs centred, the inner ankle bones go back, the outer hips go back. If these two actions do not oppose and balance each other, the legs will turn, displacing themselves in the hip socket and either tightening or overstretching the sacrum and lumbar spine.

The energetic charge of the *bandhas* is also replicated in the hands and feet.

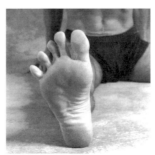

Full of life, but free from tension, hands and feet mirror the trunk: hollow at the centre, broad and full at the top, solid and stable at the bottom.

Here we have an expression of the principle that the parts reflect the whole. The base of the fingers and the ball of the foot reflect, support and resonate with the chest. The heel of both foot and hand reflect, support and resonate with the pelvis. The arch of the foot and centre of the palm reflect, support and resonate with the

53

abdomen. When activating limbs, feet and hands in this way they act as supports to the *bandhas* in the trunk, bringing about energetic union and structural harmony in the whole of the body.

All energy moves in spirals. Therefore it should be no surprise that when looked at from a broader perspective than a single detail, it turns out that the momentum of the adjustments of alignment is spirallic. This means that to establish *Asana*, we utilize the momentum and energetics of the *bandhas* throughout the whole body, unifying it into a single structural and energetic whole: a living mandala which transforms our consciousness from linear, dualistic awareness, to *samadhi*, in which subject object and action dissolve, self and other unite, *siva* and *shakti* dissolve into the ecstasy of union: this is yoga. From this perspective we can see that the *bandhas* and alignment are one.

The *bandhas*, like the other four techniques, are not sacraments. We should approach them with an open spirit of enquiry. By using them we can see what they do, and how they do it. Then we can become creatively selective in our use of them. *Jalandhara* and *Uddiyanabandha* cannot be done in all *Asana*. To try to impose them would bring strain and even minor injury. Be sensitive and responsive to your body at all times, and you will know when and where to use them. As your practice develops you will find yourself able to establish the *bandhas* more easily in more postures and hold them for longer.

54

8

PRANAYAMA: THE QUALITY OF RHYTHM

Having carefully entered a pose on the rhythm of our breath, established the spirallic adjustments in the outer body, and elicited the energetic presence of the *bandhas*, what is there left to do? Breathe. Breathe freely. Breathe fully. Breathing is the very essence of life. Oxygen our most vital nutrient. How quickly we die without it. Yet how easily, how consistently we disregard it. Hatha Yoga however demands otherwise. However, to breathe freely and fully is not as simple as it sounds.

The natural potential of our breath has long been restricted. Few of us ever know what it means to use the full capacity of our lungs. Fewer still to use it freely, effortlessly, regularly. Tension in the throat, tension in the chest, tension in the diaphragm, tension in the abdomen all conspire to inhibit our breathing. *Pranayama* is the process of releasing our breath from those tensions. Of freeing it from the restrictions imposed by life. Of allowing it to ripen and mature into something quite different from that which we are accustomed to. Only then, when it has been fully released from the subtle tensions that restrict it, can it be used to generate and harness energy effectively.

Our breath is intimately connected to our minds: to our feelings and our thoughts. The quality of our breathing directly reflects the quality of our mind. This relationship also works the other way. By adjusting the quality of our breathing, we can influence the state of our mind. But only if we adjust our breathing within the parameters of its available capacity. Not if we attempt to force our breathing to fit some preconceived pattern that is currently beyond it. Then we just add to the tension of our minds, and our bodies.

Freedom of the breath depends on both *asana* and *bandha*. The former releases tension from the limbs and spine, which gives stability and support to the movement of the lungs. The latter also support the spine, while at the same time broadening the chest and stabilizing and energizing the lungs and diaphragm. Because *asana* and *bandha* have such immediate, direct effect on the lungs, they indirectly bring about a transformation in our breathing. As the spine lengthens, the ribs open and the diaphragm and lungs stabilize, both inhalation and exhalation naturally flow more freely and more fully. By bringing clear, open attention to the flow of our breath, through the agency of *Jalandharabandha* it naturally slows down and becomes smoother, more consistent. There is no need to try to impose slowness, smoothness or fullness on the lungs. If we do we just add unnecessary tension to that with which we already have to contend.

During practice the quality of our breathing will inevitably vary. Those postures in which we are able to establish the *bandhas* and stabilize the anatomical body will produce slow, smooth, soft but potent breathing. Those postures which we are still challenged by will elicit more intense breathing. It will tend to be a little quicker, a little less smooth, and a little louder. This is normal and should be of no concern. Just as the posture is challenging your body so also it is challenging your breathing. By keeping your attention on the quality of your breathing you will find that even here it will slow down, become smoother and quieter. The problem is often simply that the challenge of a difficult posture distracts us from the breath. We become over-focused on our anatomical activity at the price of our physiological activity. But the former depends upon the latter. The muscles must have a consistent, sure supply of oxygen.

Ujjayi Breathing

Breathing with the agency of the *bandhas* is *Ujjayi pranayama*. This is the most simple *pranayama*, and is characterized by the audible sound of the breath. This sound comes from the rubbing of the breath against the throat, which can be felt all the way down into the lungs. This rubbing is a direst result of *Jalandharabandha* combined with *Uddiyanabandha* and *Mulabandha*. *Jalandhara* creates resistance in the throat, so the breath not only slows down, but makes stronger contact with the throat. This produces sound. The quality of that sound, its rhythm, consistency and power originate in the action of *Uddiyana* and *Mulabandha*. When the three *bandhas* are mature their combined effect is *Ujjayi pranayama*.

There is no need to force the breath in or out fast or hard. The harsh sound that results from this is quite different from that of *ujjayi*. The sound of *ujjayi* in itself is designed to induce tranquillity and internalization of awareness. A loud, harsh sound simply creates tension and a drain of energy. That the sound of *ujjayi* increases during difficult postures is a natural occurrence that stops when that posture is no longer difficult. The sound of a mature and refined *ujjayi* is smooth, consistent, soothing and rhythmic, with a subtle power that comes from these qualities. The power of *ujjayi* comes, not from its volume, but its quality. Not from forcing, but from the *bandhas*. To think that yoga is about quantity, whether as volume in *pranayama*, or range of movement in *asana*, is a hindrance. Quality of action and awareness, not quantity, is the touchstone of yoga practice.

Abdominal Breathing

Because so many people hold tension in the abdomen, abdominal breathing is often equated with being relaxed. Relatively speaking it might be. However, Hatha Yoga goes deeper than that relativity. To release the full potential of our body, breath and mind, we must breathe fully. This depends on freeing ourselves from all tension. Even while we still carry restricting tension, the way that we breathe can help this process of release. Abdominal breathing however is inadequate to this process. It does not allow us to challenge the more subtle and deeply embedded tension in the upper respiratory muscles. In order to do this we cannot allow the abdomen to puff out, nor even to remain passive.

The Lower Abdomen: Mulabandha

The lower abdomen must be used to stabilize the lungs and diaphragm, so that when the ribcage lifts to allow inhalation, the lungs remain anchored and are stretched and opened by the lifting of the ribs. Otherwise the lungs are lifted up with the ribs instead of stretched, and cannot open fully. By engaging the pubic abdomen in *Mulabandha* the lungs are stabilized. During inhalation this exerts some pressure on the abdominal organs, which create a gentle resistance to movement of the diaphragm. This resistance not only challenges the diaphragm to engage more fully, but also increases the pressure differential between the abdominal and thoracic cavity which further stimulates the influx of air.

Inhalation

Inhalation, then, is initiated in the pubic abdomen, by *Mulabandha*. It is continued by *Uddiyana*, through the lengthening of the abdomen, the broadening, lifting and charging of the ribcage that it elicits. The inhalation is then felt as a double helix starting just above the navel and expanding on each side out from the centre line, round to the

back of the body, to the spinal column and thence back towards the breastbone, and then on up in the same manner. This double helix starts with a broadening of the ribcrests, all the way round to the spine. As this rises it continues up the fixed ribs, to the collarbones, armpits and base of the throat. The base of the throat, which opens slightly through *Jalandhara*, while the upper throat narrows, is sucking the air in: *Jalandharabandha* supporting the action of *Mulabandha* and *Uddiyanabandha*, creating *ujjayi*.

Exhalation

Exhaling is a natural reflex, and requires no conscious initiation. It happens when your body is ready. Our part is to almost resist it. Not to stop it from happening, but to make it conscious, which tends to slow it down. We initiate this from the throat: *Jalandhara*. We use the narrowness of the upper throat to challenge the exhalation. This supports the activity of the respiratory muscles, allowing them to release more slowly, smoothly and deliberately. Other than that we simply let the exhalation go. The action of *Jalandhara*, *Uddiyana* and *Mulabandha* and the presence of direct, open attention are enough to support slow, smooth, deep exhalation.

Quality of the Breath

The quality of our breathing during *Asana* is vital. It is a gauge of the quality of our practice. If we are struggling it tells us so. If we are forcing ourselves it tells us so. If we are trying to impose something we are not ready for it tells us so. If we are not here, it tells us so. If we are calm, centred, alert and sensitive, it tells us so. Therefore we can use it as a compass to steer a course between over-enthusiasm and complacency, between force and timidity, between thoughtlessness and too much thought. It can help us to find the wave of effortless effort, calm alertness, the subtle vitality that takes us deeper into ourselves.

Our breathing should be soft, smooth, effortless, vital, rhythmic and consistent. It should not be harsh, jerky, strained, forced, uneven and inconsistent. If it is, realign your attention less on your anatomical muscles and more on the *bandhas*. Do not try to completely fill or completely empty your lungs. Let them find their own volume. Do not try to make your breath very slow. Let it find its own pace. Do not try to make it potent. Let it find its own power. The sound of your breath should be soft, but containing a subtle power. More like the wash of Mediterranean waves on sand, than the breaking of waves upon the Atlantic shore. Never hold your breath. Let it flow freely. Often we hold our breath when deeply challenged in a posture. Do not support this. Breathe out, and you will go deeper.

Observe whether exhalation or inhalation is easier for you. This will vary from posture to posture, practice to practice. One may be slower, longer, deeper, easier than the other. Don't try to force the other to imitate it. Simply give it more attention. It will respond according to its capacity. Its capacity will develop with practice.

Remember that the quality of your breath is more important than the quantity of your movement. If your breath is smooth, calm, soft and consistent those qualities will suffuse your mind also. Let your breathing fill your mind with calm, clear alertness, rather than allowing your mind to impose its anxieties and tensions on your breathing.

The Postures of Dynamic Yoga

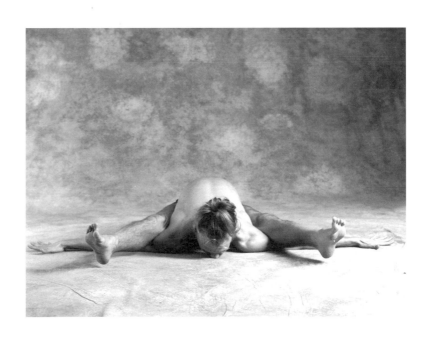

PRACTICAL CONSIDERATIONS

1. INJURIES

If you have any existing injuries, please consult a medical practitioner familiar with Hatha Yoga. Many old injuries will not hinder your practice at all, and may even be relieved by it. Others will require that you modify your practice to accommodate them. If you cannot find someone to consult, make sure you apply sensitivity to all postures affecting the injured area.

2. ILLNESS

Many illnesses can be helped through judicious Hatha Yoga. The passive, finishing sequences in particular boost vitality and enable recovery. When you are tired and debilitated by illness be careful with the more dynamic aspect of the practice. Temporary, circumstantial conditions, such as hangover, however, can be helped by a strong, dynamic practice.

If you have any of the following conditions be sure to consult a medical professional before commencing Hatha Yoga:

- multiple sclerosis
- epilepsy
- HIV or AIDS
- coronary disease
- cancer
- eye problems
- high blood pressure
- neck problems
- knee problems.

This is not because in the case of such conditions Hatha Yoga is contra-indicated. Rather that with direct guidance it can be extremely beneficial.

3. PREGNANCY

Pregnancy can be greatly enhanced by Hatha Yoga. If unable to find a specialist teacher, please consult the book *Preparing for Pregnancy through Hatha Yoga* by Janet Balaskas.

4. EATING

Please practise on an empty stomach. Allow three hours after a meal, one hour after a very light snack. Coffee or black tea just before practice can disturb the stomach and nerves. Milk will dull your sensitivity. Herbal or twig tea is fine.

5. SURFACES

Practise on a non-slip surface. Wooden and stone floors provide adequate grip. Specialist yoga mats can be very useful. Make sure that the surface you are using is flat: especially if outdoors. This is especially important for standing poses and inversions.

6. CLOTHING

The more your skin can breathe, the better. Wear as little clothing as possible. Be sure to support those parts of your anatomy that require it! Whatever you may wear should not restrict your movement, nor your blood flow: no tight waistlines or heavy materials. Wear no jewellery.

7. DRAUGHTS

Whether inside or out, do not practise in a draught. As your body warms up from the inside, which will take longer, the contrasting coolness of a draught can traumatize your muscles into tightening suddenly. Never practise under a fan, or in air-conditioning.

8. HEATING

If you are in a cold climate, or cold season, make sure your practice space is warm. Ensure that your heat source is not consuming all the available oxygen supply. Do not overheat the air around you. You will sweat excessively, without needing to develop internal heat: the sweat will represent a draining action rather than a purifying one. If you are practising in a hot room and becoming exhausted, try turning the heat down.

9. SWEATING

A little, regular sweat is healthy. Too much can be draining. The sweat should be generated by your internal activity, not your domestic heating system. It should act as insulation, keeping the heat that your activity produces inside. If your sweat is pouring off you, turn down the heat, or slow down, or both. Do not wipe the sweat from your face or body. Learn to produce enough sweat to insulate you, and not too much.

10. DURATION

Yoga postures are meant to be held. In the beginning you may have to count breaths to stay long enough to overcome your initial resistance to the poses. Another method you can use for postures which are not physically taxing is to resist coming out the first two times you think of it, leaving on the third one. When you become free in the pose you will know when to come out. It is not a question of time, but quality. Eventually you will learn how to die in a pose. Happy Birthday.

11. DISCOMFORT, SHOCK AND PAIN

Pain should neither be avoided, nor indulged. It is a part of life, it is a part of yoga. In your practice you will come across three kinds of pain.

The first, more *discomfort* than pain, is the aching discomfort of sleeping tissues being awakened. Tight muscles and connective tissue will complain as you awaken them. This is unavoidable.

63

But it should not reach a point of intrusive intensity. This means you are overstretching and damaging body tissues. Rather it should be a bearable, even pleasant aching that is in direct proportion to your movement. If you back off a little it retreats also; if you push on it intensifies. There should be a sense of relief within it, resulting from the fact that you are giving freedom back to restricted tissues.

The second, more *shock* than pain, is more sudden. It tends to be intense and without warning. The postures restructure muscular relationships, breaking down old patterns of imbalance. Many of these imbalanced patterns were established to cushion and mask injuries that were not dealt with. If you have any old injuries, or even current ones, the postures may awaken them as your body releases itself from its compensatory patterns. This kind of pain is usually not only sudden but momentary: it is gone almost as soon as it occurs. But it can be followed by painless sensations of pulling, tearing or even ripping. Again these sensations bring with them a sense of relief, as an old, limiting pattern is broken down. If you are not put off by the sudden shock you will find no difficulty in continuing your practice. It is not uncommon for experiences of this kind to occur in a particular part of your body in a number of adjacent practice sessions. When the old, restrictive muscle patterns are completely dissolved this will stop. Then you will find that you have greater and easier movement than you had before.

The third is quite definitely *pain*. If the sense of relief is not there then you must be careful, you are experiencing intrusive pain. It may be that the movement you are making is adding to an existing problem, or it may be that it is creating one. Hopefully, if you practise with sensitivity you will not experience an injury being incurred through abuse of your body. However if you are absent-minded, grasping or superficial in your practice you may do. If you do experience sudden, intense pain

that remains or intensifies, release the movement or action you have just made: slowly and carefully, making sure that your body is stable and your mind absolutely focused on what you are doing. Do not pull back impulsively, you may worsen the situation. Make sure that your withdrawal is well supported by the rest of your body. You should be able to continue with other poses, but if you cannot, end with some time sitting still, tuning in to the affected area, and then *Savasana*. Consult someone with a knowledge of anatomical restructuring and yoga to advise you how to proceed. Many medical professionals do not have this kind of knowledge. They therefore tend to play it safe by recommending complete rest. This is rarely appropriate, and can often make things worse. No movement is just avoiding the problem. The right movement in the right way must be found. Very often it is the very movement which hurts us that, if done with the correct support, heals us.

12. PRIDE

Be careful not to cultivate pride. The effect of Hatha Yoga on your body can be so pleasantly profound it can easily snare you into attachment to appearances. Once caught in that it will be at the price of sensitivity and honesty. The groundless pride of a physically adept yoga student is a sad and demeaning result of superficial practice.

13. AMBITION

Equally take care not to be driven by ambition. It also will diminish your sensitivity and honesty. You might be convinced that if you can just balance on your head for an hour, or on one finger for a minute, or wrap your legs around your neck, or place the back of your head on your buttocks, you will no longer suffer from the anxieties and uncertainties that you long to escape. Not so. There is no magical escape from yourself. Your fears and doubts, your sense of inadequacy or unhappiness cannot be erased by the mastery of magical techniques, or the ritualistic repetition of mystical rites. Yoga is not cloud-cuckoo land. The only way to free yourself from your limitations is to face them, not escape them. Practise yoga with an open heart and it will reward you. Practise it with the anxious grip of a grasping mind and it will bind you further.

14. ATTITUDE

Just as important as what you are doing are how you are doing it and why. Our actions and their effects are coloured by our intentions, attitude and feelings. This is as true for those that are unconscious as conscious. If you approach your practice with the sole intention of reaching a predetermined goal, you run a great risk. That is of ignoring yourself, your feelings, your capabilities, your limits, your needs, just as you are. All sacrificed on the sanctified altar of your desires. But in the end there is nothing for you to find other than yourself. No matter how long you spend chasing the wild geese of noble aspirations, if they are not a part of who and what you are you will be lost in the chase. But, if you simply set out to find out, exhaustively, who and what you are you may find that you are something more brilliant and wonderful than anything you may have heard or dreamed of.

15. EMOTIONAL DISCHARGE

If you go deep enough into the physical patterns of your body, you will uncover underlying emotional blocks. In doing so you will disturb them: dislodge them from their nests. You then have the opportunity to resolve and release them: by turning the light of your stable, open, full, direct awareness upon them. This you need to do if you begin to feel any emotional disturbance as you enter the 'tha', finishing part of your practice. Especially when you are sitting still, or lying in *Savasana*, any emotional release will surface. Allow it to do so. Do not fight it. Do not displace your awareness into fantasy. Be

present, and allow it to resolve itself in the light of your attention. These feelings can include anger, grief, lust, shame, regret, fear, anxiety, sorrow, despair, etc. Do not attribute these feelings directly to the practice itself: it is only bringing them into the foreground. Do not think that you should not be feeling them. You are. They are not wrong. They are part of you in this moment.

However, be aware that imbalanced practice can create its own unnecessary disturbances. This can be the result of forcing your muscles in a pose, pushing yourself to continue beyond your actual capacity, moving too quickly in or out of poses and too fast between them, subjugating your breath to either your body or your mind, insensitivity, greed, fear or pride. The most common feeling that this creates is anger: and its progeny, impatience, intolerance, criticism, cynicism and nihilism. It results from your being insensitive and aggressive to yourself. Don't.

16. PHYSICAL DISCHARGE

Hatha Yoga can also precipitate physical discharge. This is part of its purifying, detoxifying effect. Do not be alarmed if you find skin eruptions, rashes, diarrhoea, ear or nose discharge, following your practice. This is simply a sign of an imbalanced diet/lifestyle now being compensated for in your practice. If it persists consult someone with training in the natural care of the body as part of the body/mind continuum.

17. REGULARITY

A little and often is more beneficial than a lot occasionally. You may practise every day, although occasional rests will often stimulate greater progress when you resume. Variety in your practice will be more beneficial than always practising in the same way. This can be done even using the same posture sequence, by varying the emphasis: focusing on alignment, or on *vinyasa*, or on the *bandhas* or on breathing or on awareness, or any combination thereof. Some Indian teachers recommend not practising on the full moon, some also not on the new moon. Because of the energetics of these times especial care must be taken in any practice that you do.

18. REMINDERS
Remember always to:

- keep your weight even across your foundation
- keep your hands and feet alive
- use your arms and legs to support the energy of the *bandhas*
- align your pelvis so that it connects your legs and spine freely
- maintain the *bandhas* so your abdomen is long, hollow and passive, your chest broad, full and active
- maintain the line of your neck as an extension of the spine unless you are deliberately taking the chin up or down
- adjust your body and *bandhas* so that your breath is as free, smooth, soft and rhythmic as possible
- let your breathing guide your body, and allow your body to accommodate your breathing
- remain aware of exactly what you are doing, and how that affects the whole of your body
- feel all of the changing sensations inside you just as they arise, without judgement
- use your constant awareness of changing sensations to guide you deeper into your body and mind
- enjoy your practice, enjoy yourself.

10

THE PRACTICE OF SURYANAMASKAR AND VINYASA

Traditionally Hatha Yoga practice begins with a sequence known as the Sun Salutation. This warms up the body, awakens the breathing, initiates breath/body synchronization, focuses the mind and prepares for the posture practice. Where Sun Salutations are indicated in the Foundation and Preparatory series, repeat until you are warm, focused, soft and ready for the standing poses. There is no need to count. You may rest in Dog Pose during Sun Salutations if you wish, but this is not obligatory.

In order to ensure muscular compensation and preparation, to maintain the free rhythm of our breathing, to allow for a recentring of body mind and energy, to develop heat, concentration and deep internalization the postures are connected by a *vinyasa* sequence. This is always done on the breath, so that each movement synchronizes with either the exhalation or the inhalation. Dog Pose is sometimes held to rest and centre in. The traditional *Vinyasas* are based on the Sun Salutation. Start by using *Sukhavinyasa* (see page 74), then progress to the *Vinyasa* (page 79). When tired you can use *Svanavinyasa* (page 76) or *Sukhullola* (page 77).

Vinyasa do not have to be used to connect the standing postures, nor the inverted postures, but feel free to do so if you wish. Give yourself the chance to truly understand the function and benefits of the *Vinyasa* by experimenting with using different ones in different ways at different times. Invent your own, always remembering breath/body synchronization, inhaling when the front of the body opens and exhaling when it closes.

In the Pacifying Series no specific *Vinyasa* is indicated. Simply find the easiest, simplest way from one pose to the next incurring the least distraction and use of energy. Once you are comfortable with a *vinyasa* you may insert it if you wish.

Sukhasuryanamaskar

Sukhasuryanamaskar is learned and used in the Foundation Series. The postures are not held. Each movement from one posture to the next is synchronized exactly with either the inhalation or exhalation as indicated.

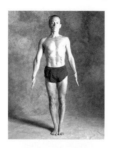

Step 1. Exhale in *Tadasana*
Stand upright, feet together, energize the trunk, legs, feet, arms and hands, looking straight ahead.

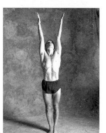

Step 2. Inhale to *Urdhvahastasana*
Raise the arms alongside the ears, looking between the palms above the head, maintaining the charge in the trunk, legs, feet, arms and hands.

70

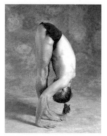

Step 3. Exhale to *Uttanasana*
Pivot the pelvis and, keeping the charge in legs and feet, extend the spine along the legs, head towards the ankles, keeping the abdomen long, hollow and empty, palms to the floor or hands on the ankles or shins.

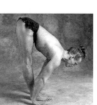

Step 4. Inhale to *Ardhuttanasana*
Keeping the charge in feet, legs and trunk, extend the spine forwards and raise the head, keeping the abdomen long, hollow and empty.

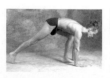 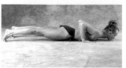

Step 5. Exhale and step/jump to *Ardhachaturangadandasana*
Taking the legs back as far as you can, feet hip-width apart, bend the arms and bring the chest to the floor with the elbows above the wrists and the legs strong; the abdomen, pelvis and legs off the floor.

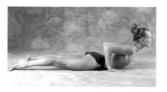

Step 6. Inhale to *Ardhurdhvamukhasvanasana*

Slip the toes back, tops of the feet and legs onto the floor and, with the legs strong, press with the hands and raise the chest and head, looking forwards, keeping the abdomen and pelvis on the floor as well as the legs and feet.

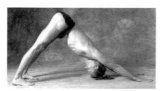

Step 7. Exhale to *Adhomukhasvanasana*

Pushing from the hands, roll over the toes and raise the hips straight up, head and chest going down, and push the body into a V-shape, hands and feet only on the floor. Hold if you wish.

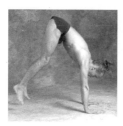

Step 8. Inhale and step/jump to *Ardhuttanasana*

Bring both legs forwards feet between the hands, feet together, legs strong. Extend the spine forwards and look up with the abdomen long, hollow and empty.

71

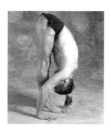

Step 9. Exhale to *Uttanasana*

Keeping the charge in the feet and legs, extend the spine along the legs, head towards the ankles, keeping the abdomen long, hollow and empty, palms to the floor or hands on the ankles or shins.

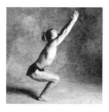

Step 10. Inhale to *Utktasana*

Bend the legs while raising the trunk and arms, palms together, and look up along the arms.

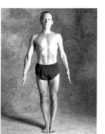

Step 11. Exhale to *Tadasana*

Straighten the legs while bringing the palms down to the sides, arms still straight and strong, legs, feet and hands alive.

Suryanamaskar

Suryanamaskar is used to start off the Preparatory Series. The postures are not held. Each movement from one posture to the next is synchronized exactly with either the inhalation or exhalation as indicated.

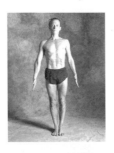

Step 1. Exhale in *Tadasana*
Stand upright, feet together, energize the trunk, legs, feet, arms and hands, looking straight ahead.

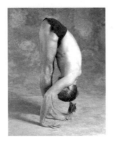

Step 2. Inhale to *Urdhvahastasana*
Raise the arms alongside the ears, looking between the palms above the head, maintaining the charge in the trunk, legs, feet, arms and hands.

72

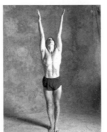

Step 3. Exhale to *Uttanasana*
Pivot the pelvis and, keeping the charge in legs and feet, extend the spine along the legs, head towards the ankles, keeping the abdomen long, hollow and empty, palms to the floor or hands on the ankles or shins.

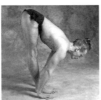

Step 4. Inhale to *Ardhuttanasana*
Keeping the charge in feet, legs and trunk, extend the spine forwards and raise the head, keeping the abdomen long, hollow and empty.

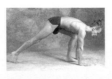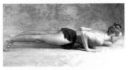

Step 5. Exhale and step/jump to *Chaturangadandasana*
Taking the legs back as far as you can, feet hip-width apart, bend the arms and bring the legs and trunk parallel to the floor with the elbows above the wrists and the legs strong, only the hands and balls of the feet on the floor.

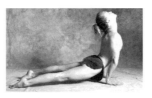

Step 6. Inhale to *Urdhvamukhasvanasana*
Roll forwards on to the tops of the feet, front ankles long and, with the legs strong and kept off the floor, press with the hands and raise the chest and head, keeping the pelvis close to the floor with the tops of the feet on the floor, front ankle long, hands, ankles and feet only on the floor.

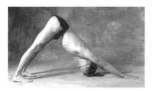

Step 7. Exhale to *Adhomukhasvanasana*
Pushing from the hands, roll over the toes and raise the hips straight up, head and chest going down, and push the body into a V-shape, hands and feet only on the floor. Hold if you wish.

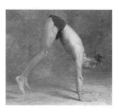
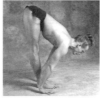

Step 8. Inhale and step/jump to *Ardhuttanasana*
Bring both legs forwards, feet between the hands, feet together, legs strong. Extend the spine forwards and look up with the abdomen long, hollow and empty.

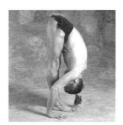

73

Step 9. Exhale to *Uttanasana*
Keeping the charge in the feet and legs, extend the spine along the legs, head towards the ankles, keeping the abdomen long, hollow and empty, palms to the floor or hands on the ankles or shins.

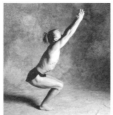

Step 10. Inhale to *Utktasana*
Bend the legs while raising the trunk and arms, palms together, and look up along the arms.

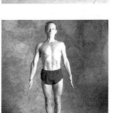

Step 11. Exhale to *Tadasana*
Straighten the legs while bringing the palms down to the sides, arms still straight and strong, legs, feet and hands alive.

Sukhavinyasa

Sukhavinyasa is used in between floor postures, or each side of a floor posture when in the Foundation Series. The postures are not held. Each movement from one posture to the next is synchronized exactly with either the inhalation or exhalation as indicated.

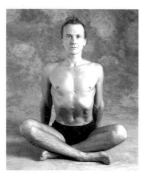

Step 1. Exhale to *Sukhasana*
Crossing the legs easily in front of you while remaining on the buttocks.

74

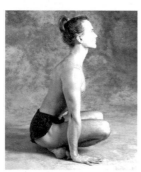

Step 2. Inhale to *Urdhvasukhasana*
Bring the arms round the shins, palms to the floor, and bring the weight forward off the buttocks and onto the feet and palms, looking straight ahead.

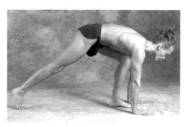

Step 3. Exhale and step/jump to *Ardhachaturangadandasana*
Taking the legs back as far as you can, feet hip-width apart, bend the arms and bring the chest to the floor with the elbows above the wrists and the legs strong; abdomen, pelvis and legs off the floor.

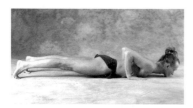

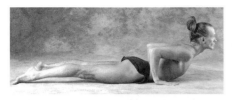

Step 4. Inhale to *Ardhurdhvamukhasvanasana*

Slip the toes back, tops of the feet and legs onto the floor and, with the legs strong, press with the hands and raise the chest and head, keeping the abdomen and pelvis on the floor along with the legs and feet.

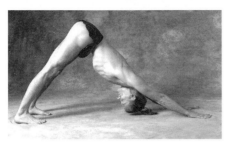

Step 5. Exhale to *Adhomukhasvanasana*

Pressing with the palms, roll over the toes, raise the hips straight up, head and chest going down, and push the body into a V-shape, hands and feet only on the floor. Hold if you wish.

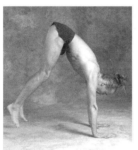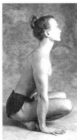

Step 6. Inhale and step/jump to *Urdhvasukhasana*

Bring the arms round the shins, palms to the floor, and bring the weight forward off the buttocks and onto the feet and palms, looking straight ahead.

75

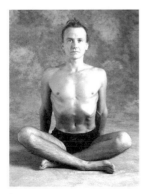

Step 7. Exhale to *Sukhasana*

Roll back on to the buttocks.

Svanavinyasa

Svanavinyasa is used in between floor postures, or each side of a floor posture when feeling too tired to do other *vinyasa*. The postures are not held. Each movement from one posture to the next is synchronized exactly with either the inhalation or exhalation as indicated.

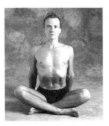

Step 1. Exhale to *Sukhasana*
Crossing the legs easily in front of you while remaining on the buttocks.

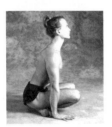

Step 2. Inhale to *Urdhvasukhasana*
Bring the arms round the shins, palms to the floor, and bring the weight forward off the buttocks and onto the feet and palms, looking straight ahead.

76

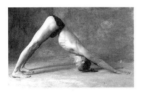

Step 3. Exhale to *Adhomukhasvanasana*
Pressing with the palms, take the feet back hip-width apart, raise the hips straight up, head and chest going down, and push the body into a V-shape, hands and feet only on the floor. Hold if you wish.

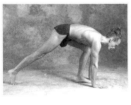

Step 4. Inhale and step/jump to *Urdhvasukhasana*
Bring the arms round the shins, palms to the floor, and bring the weight forward off the buttocks and onto the feet and palms, looking straight ahead.

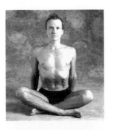

Step 5. Exhale to *Sukhasana*
Roll back on to the buttocks.

Sukhullola

Sukhullola is used in between floor postures, or each side of a floor posture when feeling too tired to do *Svanavinyasa*. The postures are not held. Each movement from one posture to the next is synchronized exactly with either the inhalation or exhalation as indicated.

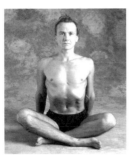

Step 1. Exhale to *Sukhasana*
Crossing the legs easily in front of you while remaining on the buttocks.

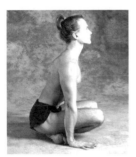

Step 2. Inhale to *Urdhvasukhasana*
Bring the arms round the shins, palms to the floor, and bring the weight forward off the buttocks and onto the feet and palms, looking straight ahead.

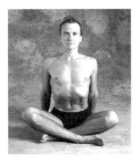

Step 3. Exhale to *Sukhasana*
Roll back on to the buttocks.

77

Svanullola

Svanullola is used to connect two poses that are done lying on the front of the body. This is only the case towards the end of the Foundation Series, between *Ardhurdhvamukhasvanasana* (Posture No. 13) and *Urdhvamukhasvanasana* (Posture No. 14), *vinyasas* not being used in the Pacifying Series. The postures are not held. Each movement from one posture to the next is synchronized exactly with either the inhalation or exhalation as indicated.

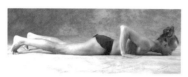

Step 1. Inhale
Rest the whole body on the floor, toes tucked in hip-width apart and palms behind the armpits, wrists under the elbows.

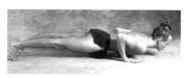

Step 2. Exhale to *Chaturangadandasana*
Feet hip-width apart, bring the hands behind the armpits with the elbows above the wrists, press with the palms and bring the legs and trunk parallel to the floor with the legs strong, only the hands and balls of the feet on the floor.

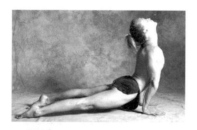

Step 3. Inhale to *Urdhvamukhasvanasana*
Roll forwards onto the tops of the feet, front ankle long and with the legs strong and kept off the floor. Press with the hands and raise the chest and head, keeping the pelvis close to the floor with the tops of the feet on the floor, front ankle long, hands, ankles and feet only on the floor.

78

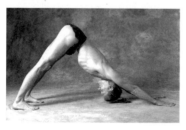

Step 4. Exhale to *Adhomukhasvanasana*
Pushing from the hands, roll back over the toes and raise the hips straight up, head and chest going down, and push the body into a V-shape, hands and feet only on the floor. Hold if you wish.

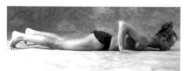

Step 5. Inhale
Drop the front of the body to floor.

Vinyasa

The *Vinyasa* is used to connect the floor poses of the Preparatory Series. This does not include the standing or inverted poses. It is not only done between postures, but also between each side of poses done for each leg. The postures are not held. Each movement from one posture to the next is synchronized exactly with either the inhalation or exhalation as indicated.

Step 1. Exhale to *Sukhasana*
Crossing the legs easily in front of you while remaining on the buttocks.

Step 2. Inhale to *Urdhvasukhasana*
Bring the arms round the shins, palms to the floor, and bring the weight forward off the buttocks and onto the feet and palms, looking straight ahead.

Step 3. Exhale and step/jump to *Chaturangadandasana*
Taking the legs back as far as you can, feet hip-width apart, bend the arms and bring the legs and trunk parallel to the floor with the elbows above the wrists and the legs strong, only the hands and balls of the feet on the floor.

79

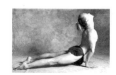

Step 4. Inhale to *Urdhvamukhasvanasana*
Roll forwards onto the tops of the feet, front ankle long and with the legs strong and kept off the floor. Press with the hands and raise the chest and head, keeping the pelvis close to the floor with the tops of the feet on the floor, front ankle long, hands, ankles and feet only on the floor.

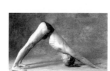

Step 5. Exhale to *Adhomukhasvanasana*
Pushing from the hands, roll over the toes and raise the hips straight up, head and chest going down, and push the body into a V-shape, hands and feet only on the floor. Hold if you wish.

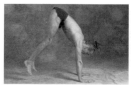

Step 6. Inhale and step/jump to *Urdhvasukhasana*
Bring the arms round the shins, palms to the floor, and bring the weight forward off the buttocks and onto the feet and palms, looking straight ahead.

Step 7. Exhale to *Sukhasana*
Roll back on to the buttocks.

Vinyasana

Vinyasana is the dynamic practice of one *asana*, or two *asana* in combination. It allows the body and mind to go deeper without force, as they soften and open through the act of repetition. The following three *Vinyasana* are used at the beginning of the Foundation Series. They can, however, be used any time any of their postures is indicated.

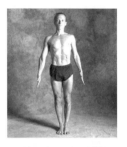

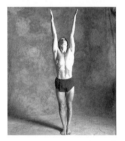

Urdhvahastullola
Alternate between the following two movements until they are effortlessly synchronized with their inhalation and exhalations.

> From *Tadasana*
> **Inhale** to *Urdhvahastasana*
> raise the arms alongside the ears, looking at the palms as they face each other or touch above the head, maintaining a charge in the trunk, legs, feet, arms and hands.
> **Exhale** to *Tadasana*
> bring the head down to look straight ahead as you bring the palms back to the thighs – feet, legs, arms, hands and trunk alive.

80

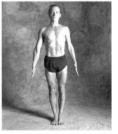

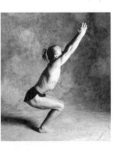

Utktullola
Alternate between the following two movements until they are effortlessly synchronized with their inhalation and exhalations.

> From *Tadasana*
> **Inhale** to *Utktasana*
> bend the legs while raising the trunk and arms, palms together, and look up along the arms.
> **Exhale** to *Tadasana*
> straighten the legs while bringing the palms down to the sides, arms still straight and strong, legs, feet and hands alive.

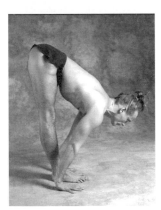

Uttanullola

Alternate between the following two movements until they are
effortlessly synchronized with their inhalation and exhalations.

From *Uttanasana*
Inhale to *Ardhuttanasana*
keeping the charge in the feet, legs and trunk, extend the spine
forwards and raise the head, keeping the abdomen long, hollow
and empty.
Exhale to *Uttanasana*
keeping the charge in the legs and feet, extend the spine along
the legs, head towards the ankles, keeping the abdomen long,
hollow and empty, palms to the floor or hands on the ankles or
shins.

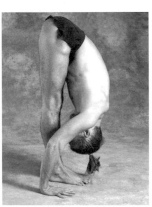

81

11

THE POSTURES

There is much more to a yoga posture than simply making a shape in space. Although many of those shapes are familiar from observation of gymnastics, sports, dance and children playing, that familiarity is superficial. Yoga involves a use of the muscles that is quite different from that of other activities. Usually we utilize muscle contraction to elicit a physical action. Muscles that lengthen do so to balance those contractions. In yoga it is the opposite. Our intention is to lengthen the muscles: contractions are utilized to support and balance this process. However, it is important to remember that Hatha Yoga is not an esoteric form of stretching. Although Hatha Yoga does result in flexibility, that is not its goal, simply a by-product. Going for maximum movement in a yoga posture misses the whole point, and can result in weakening of muscles, joints and tendons and in muscular and nervous imbalance. The stretching that occurs in yoga has three purposes. One to compensate for tight muscles. Two to create space in and between the joints. Three, and most important, to bring about a change in the state of the nervous system. By forcing the stretch we may initiate new areas of tension, de-stabilize the joints, and overstimulate the nervous system.

Our muscles are usually either in a state of contraction, compensatory extension, or residual tone. Residual tone is when we experience a muscle as being relaxed. However it is still being fed nervous impulses. These impulses ensure that when a command to contract arrives the muscle fibres will immediately respond. In other words, the muscle is not entirely relaxed. Given the fact that we also have residual *tension* in many of our muscles, not using a muscle is not necessarily a restful condition. Residual tone and residual tension mean that our sensory motor nervous system is constantly under pressure, even when we are asleep. It is one of the functions of Hatha Yoga to access the energy and potential of the central nervous system. When the sensory motor nervous system is truly at rest, this becomes more possible. The yoga postures, then, are designed not just to release residual tension, implanted in the muscles from a lifetime's stress and strain, but also to reduce residual tone: bringing them into a deeper state of relaxation. When all of the muscles in the body are able to relax, to give up their activity, however subtle it may have been, then the sensory motor nervous system can rest. This means that, due to the fact that our senses and motor muscles form a single continuum, our senses also rest. Our attention, then, is drawn away from our motor muscles and our senses, towards our central nervous system. This is the beginning of the process of sense withdrawal, or internalization of awareness so basic to the aims of Hatha Yoga.

The postures described in this section are utilized in sequences. Traditionally each posture has not only its own inherent form, but also a specific mode of entering and leaving, and also its place in a sequence of postures that ensures that it is adequately prepared and compensated for. The instructions for each posture include how to enter and leave it, the basic shape and subtle adjustments of the pose, its effects and purposes. Even the most basic posture can result in muscular strain if not approached in the right way. Therefore, take great care if you decide to do any posture in isolation. Be sure that you do not force yourself, and that you listen to the feedback of your body, rather than being carried away by the enthusiasm of your mind and its desires and intentions.

There is no greater safeguard in yoga than sensitive, honest awareness. To push yourself beyond your limits will reduce and not expand them. Rather, bring yourself gently to your current limit, and stay there a while: then your limits will naturally and easily expand. But remember that each day is new, and your capacity of yesterday may not be available today. Perhaps you did not sleep well. Perhaps you are preoccupied or in a hurry. Your mind can reduce your capacity just as easily as your body can. Stay aware.

Each posture has a Sanskrit name. Many of the Sanskrit names are made up of words that describe them. Some are named after ancient yogis. Sanskrit is the mother of many contemporary languages. It has certain qualities English does not. One is that it is very flexible and dynamic. A word does not have a single, fixed meaning. The exact meaning of a Sanskrit word depends on where and how it is used: on its context. This gives it a remarkable range of expressiveness. It also makes it a little difficult for Westerners with a static view of language to navigate. The names of the poses have a vibrational resonance with the postures and their effect. They are therefore useful to learn. Many students find that simply saying the name of a pose can facilitate its performance. Translations of Sanskrit words are given in the glossary. Pronunciation is complex. The most important thing to remember that there is no hard 'a' as in hat. *Asana* is pronounced aahsuhnuh: Sanskrit 'a' being either aah or uh. Emphasis is usually given to the second last syllable.

The immediate purpose of Hatha Yoga is to bring about profound relaxation on every level of our being. This, and only this, allows our full potential to ripen, our true nature to express itself unhindered. It is not simply a matter of finding the line of least resistance, without making any effort. Tension is so ubiquitous and deep inside us that we don't even notice most of it. Therefore, to make ourselves comfortable is not the same thing as relaxing. If it were, there are many easier ways than

83

yoga to relax: drink, drugs, sex, sun. However, the relaxation that these offer is superficial and momentary. They relieve us for a while of our feelings of tension, perhaps, but they are not enough to remove our tensions permanently. For this to occur a little judicious effort is required.

Effort can be of two kinds. Constructive, energizing effort, or destructive, exhausting effort. It is by applying the former to our tension that yoga permits genuine relaxation to occur. Relaxation itself cannot be imposed. Not by any amount of wishful thinking, drugs or effort. Rather, relaxation is an art. A profound and challenging one. To release ourselves permanently from residual tension, we must challenge its presence in our body. Effort must be directed towards the tensions in such a way that they dissolve, leaving us in a genuine state of relaxation. In Hatha Yoga, of course, this is done through the agency of *asana*, *vinyasa*, *bandha*, *pranayama* and *drushti*.

This means that whatever we do must not create tension. Our compass for guiding our practice so that it does not reinforce or generate tension is the core of the body. The core of the body, including the pelvic floor, the front spine, the throat, face and brain, should always be passive, relaxed, receptive. Especial care should be taken to keep the anus, navel and jaw completely relaxed. Our actions should utilize effort judiciously, until they produce a state of effortlessness. This occurs when each individual action, sustained by only that much effort that it requires, combines with all of the others to create an integrated state that feels effortless: completely stable, and completely comfortable: effortless effort. Learning the meaning of effortless effort means learning to recognize and find our edge.

To support this process we need only to apply honest sensitivity to what we are doing. This cannot occur if we are trying to reach a predetermined goal, regardless of our condition and capacity. This is a subtle form of violence that will exhaust and

84

frustrate us sooner or later. Instead we must try to approach our practice openly. As an exploration of the territory: ourselves, just as we are. It is the nature of life that that which is fully itself will change and in this change, grow. We do not have to force change on ourselves. It is inevitable. We can, however, assist or hinder it. So that it becomes growth or decay. Yoga is about learning to assist it in every aspect of our lives. It is vital, therefore, that in our yoga practice we do not hinder it, by pushing past the edge, or giving up before reaching it.

Each pose is different from all of the other ones. However there is also a unity between them. This consists of the way that we approach them, and the effect that they have on our energy, state of mind and awareness. Rather than approaching them from the surface differences, we attempt to do so from the central core. From our awareness, from our breathing, from the core of the body. Although we are utilizing muscular adjustments we orchestrate them to a more subtle theme. While entering the pose we extend our awareness out from our deepest centre into each part of the body. This creates an inner dynamic, a flow of attention and energy from the centre to the periphery. From this dynamic we utilize the muscular adjustments. The deeper the place from which you start, and the more evenly and fully you release the energy outwards, the less consideration you will have to give to muscular detail. By approaching the whole from the centre, the parts will take care of themselves. Of course, this depends upon a refined and stable quality of awareness, and an acute sensitivity to what is happening as a result of what you are doing. This takes time to flourish. Be patient. At the same time, however, we also allow our awareness of the peripheral surfaces to lead us back in to the centre. So that while we try to initiate from our centre, there is always a complementary, supporting flow of energy and awareness back in as well as out.

The key to this creative dynamic is the energetics of the *bandhas*. By energizing the whole body, from the core to the periphery the structural demands of the shape we are making will spontaneously elicit the subtle adjustments of *asana*. This requires spiralling energy in the trunk and limbs: the action of the *bandhas*. It depends upon depth of awareness. As our awareness deepens, becomes clearer, more open, more direct, we will depend less and less on our accumulable knowledge and understanding of *Asana* and its techniques, because we will be experiencing it. Then we begin to find that any pose, if it embodies *Asana*, is enough, is yoga.

How long you spend on a pose is determined by you, and varies day to day. Take your time entering with clarity, precision and sensitivity. Then take time to stay still in the pose, challenging your tension and your limits carefully and consciously. Then come out deliberately, with the same clarity, precision and sensitivity with which you entered. In the beginning you may like to count breaths in a pose, to establish a rhythm. How many depends on the length of your breath, which will vary day to day and posture to posture. However, do not become dependent on counting as a measure. It can easily become a way to evade challenging your limits honestly. Let your body, not your mind, tell you when the work in the posture that you are currently capable of has been done. It knows.

Standing postures should not be held any longer if you are shaking and cannot find any adjustment to relieve this. Nor should they be held if irresistible tension is coming anywhere into the body. Floor postures, including inversions, will give much more benefit if you stay in them longer than you feel like it. The first time you think of leaving, stay. And the second. Come out the third time. You will be less likely to be running away from the challenge the pose is presenting to your structural tensions and imposed limitations.

The yoga postures in this book have very exact relationships to each other. This depends to a great extent on the sequence of postures within which they are practised. If the postures are practised in the sequences outlined they will not only be easier to assimilate, but in combination they reinforce, enhance and deepen each other's effects. For exactly the same reason all the postures, with the exception of standing and inverted postures, should be linked by a *vinyasa* in both the Foundation and Preparatory Series. There are options for this outlined in Chapter 4. However, you will find that at any given time one *vinyasa* will work the best for you.

Obviously, then, it is important that you familiarize yourself with the vinyasa options before you practise the Foundation and Preparatory Series. Underneath the Summary and at the end of the detailed instructions for each posture the posture to be done next is indicated. The number is the Posture number, not the page number. Where a posture is used in more than one Series, the different options for the next posture are indicated by different symbols: ✴ for the Pacifying Series, ▪ for the Foundation Series, and ● for the Preparatory Series.

The Art of Relaxation

Whenever we end a session we finish in the same posture: *Savasana*. This is the most difficult posture of all. In it we simply lie absolutely still and relax. But we now no longer have or can use the techniques of *asana*, *vinyasa*, *bandha*, *pranayama*, we have only *drushti* left to support our relaxation. This makes it extremely difficult to actually let go. Instead we just drift off into a distracting haze of fantasy and reminiscence. This must be resisted, firmly but gently. Time must be given to *Savasana* to permit a smooth transition from practice to life. The effects of practice are deep and affect us on every level. Allow time for everything to settle down and find its new place: heart beat, breathing, hormones, etc. Go slowly through the body as you relax, feeling the changing sensations inside you. Giving special attention to the core of the body, allow each part of the body to relax in its own time and in its own sequence. This will not always be the same. Allow those parts which release easily and quickly to encourage and support the release of those that do not. Feel everything that occurs inside you as your body lets go, allowing your awareness to tune in to more and more subtle sensations and energies. Feel muscles softening, muscle fibres lengthening, tissues opening. Feel the breath in the nostrils, throat, lungs; feel the movement, as you breathe, of the abdomen, ribcage, vertebrae, armpits, collarbones, breastbone, groins, pelvic floor. Feel the flow of the blood; sensations of movement; pressure, temperature; change of any kind. Allow your awareness to be completely absorbed by the infinite sensations of your body letting go. Allow your body to be completely penetrated by your awareness. Until there is no part of your awareness that is not inside your body, and no part of your body that is not embraced by your awareness. As you learn to apply this quality of awareness in *Savasana* you will be able to apply it in the other *asana* also.

No. 1 Savasana

The Corpse Pose

This fundamental posture resembles a corpse, with the whole body motionless and relaxed. It is always used as the last *Asana*, and sometimes at other times also. More than any other it permits complete pacification of the core of the body. As you become familiar with *Savasana*, you will be able to release surface tension from the body very quickly and enter at will into a state of physical relaxation. It promotes a state of easy, alert restfulness: brings the mind into direct contact with the body without the distraction of activity; and directs the mind towards a meditative state.

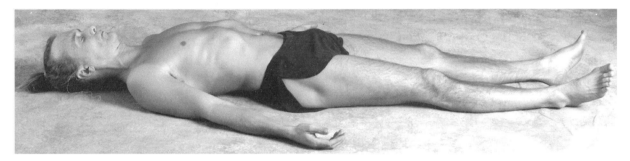

SUMMARY

Let the whole of the body sink effortlessly into itself and into the floor while you feel all of the changing sensations inside you. ✷

1 Lie flat on your back, body symmetrical, palms up with arms a little away from your body.
2 From the back of your skull, gently lengthen your neck and throat, and draw your shoulders away from your skull.
3 Lengthen your waist by drawing your buttocks away from your trunk, relaxing your lower back towards the floor, without pressing your spine down.
4 Relax your whole body into the floor, feeling your bones becoming heavier, muscles becoming lighter.
5 Become aware of the surface of your body, its contact with clothing, air and floor. Then draw that awareness inwards, cultivating a sensation of softening and melting throughout the whole of your body, until it feels light, open, at ease.

6 Feel your whole body relaxing, especially give time to relaxing the muscles of the jaw, the lower back, the pelvic floor and the abdomen.
7 Continue to allow your awareness to flow softly throughout your body from core to periphery, periphery to core: from surface to depths, depths to surface. Allow the presence of your awareness in each part of your body to encourage it to soften, to lighten, to open.

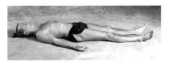

8 Continuously feel all of the changing sensations inside you as your mind softens and opens along with the whole of your body. Hold as long as you wish. ✷

No. 2 Suptahastullola

Supine Arm Wave

This is a dynamic combination of *Savasana* and *Suptahastasana* in which the arms are moved in time with the breath, flowing freely and effortlessly like a wave. It awakens the arms, hands and shoulder joints and initiates breath/body synchronization, harmonizing the activity of the anatomical and physiological bodies. It teaches the relationship between the movement of the arms and the chest and abdomen, and therefore the *bandhas*.

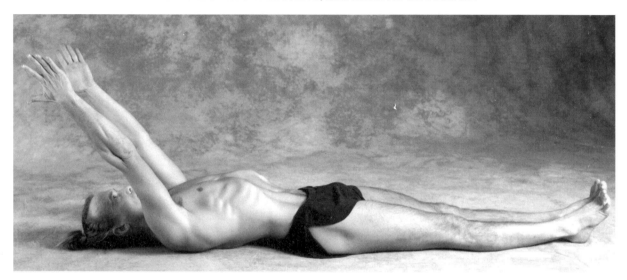

SUMMARY

Lying on the back and maintaining *Uddiyana* and *Mulabandha* while keeping the arms charged, alternately raise them past the ears as you inhale, and back again as you exhale, exactly in time with your breathing.

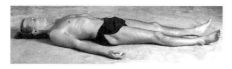

1 Lie in *Savasana*.

2 **Inhaling**, broaden your ribcrest and suck your solar plexus in and up so your chest becomes active, broad and full, your abdomen passive, long and empty (*Uddiyanabandha*), and flatten your pubic abdomen, sucking your perineum and sacrum in, with your anus soft (*Mulabandha*).

3 **Exhaling**, roll your palms down to the floor, lengthen your arms, broaden your palms and lengthen your fingers. At the same time broaden the balls of your feet, press the inner ankles together and suck the thigh muscles in so your legs become charged and straight.

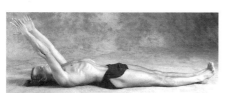

4 Maintaining the charge in your legs, feet, hands and arms, **inhale** slowly and raise your arms up and over past your ears till they reach the floor past your head. Synchronize this movement exactly with your **inhalation**.

5 Immediately **exhale** slowly and, maintaining the charge in your legs, feet, hands and arms, lower your arms back to the starting position (**2**). Synchronize this movement exactly with your **exhalation**.

6 Continue to alternate between these two movements, until they are exactly synchronous with your breathing, keeping a charge in your legs and the core of your body soft. ✪

No. 3 Suptapadullola

Supine Leg Wave

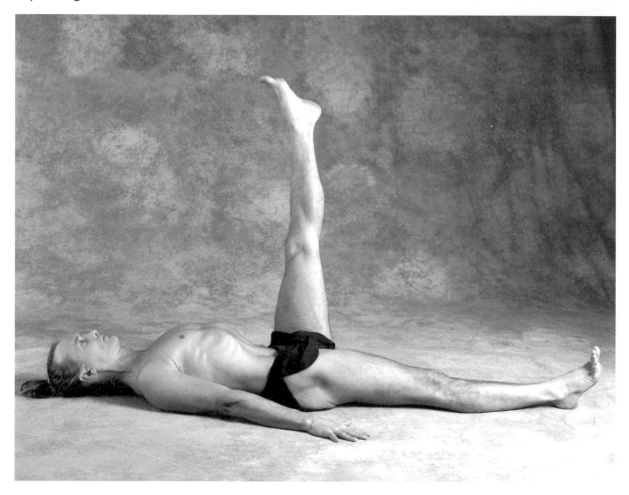

This is a dynamic combination of *Savasana* and *Suptaikapadasana*, in which the legs are moved in time with the breath, flowing freely and effortlessly like a wave. It awakens the legs, feet and hip joints and stimulates breath/body synchronization, harmonizing the activity of the anatomical and physiological bodies.

SUMMARY
Lying on the back, while maintaining *Uddiyana* and *Mulabandha*, alternately raise as you exhale, and lower as you inhale, each straight leg, exactly in time with your breathing.

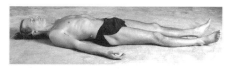

1   Lie in *Savasana*.

2   **Exhaling**, suck your thigh muscles into your legs and, broadening the balls of your feet, engage the calf muscles. At the same time lengthen your front and inner ankle and your Achilles tendon, so your foot is alive and your ankle joint evenly open.

3   **Inhaling**, broaden your ribcrest and suck your solar plexus in and up so your chest becomes active, broad and full, your abdomen passive, long and empty (*Uddiyanabandha*), and flatten your pubic abdomen, sucking your perineum in, with your anus soft (*Mulabandha*).

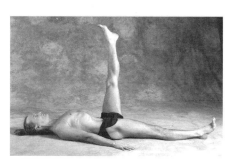

4   **Exhaling**, raise one leg straight, until it reaches its highest comfortable point exactly as your lungs become empty.

5   **Inhaling**, lower your straight leg back down to the floor so that it lands exactly when your lungs are full.

6   **Exhaling**, raise your other leg as in **4**.

7   **Inhaling**, lower your other leg as in **5**.

8   Continue to alternate between these movements, until the movement of each leg is exactly synchronous with the breathing. Keep both legs charged and straight throughout, and the core of your body soft.

91

No. 4 Bhujadhanurasana

Shoulder Bow

This pose is a dynamic one involving the whole body. It works on the spine as a gentle back bend. Care must be taken to keep the lower back soft, while giving it strong support with the feet. It establishes the use of the foundation in lifting and supporting the whole body; awakens the spine and open the chest; synchronizes body movement with breathing and harmonizes the activity of the anatomical and physiological bodies.

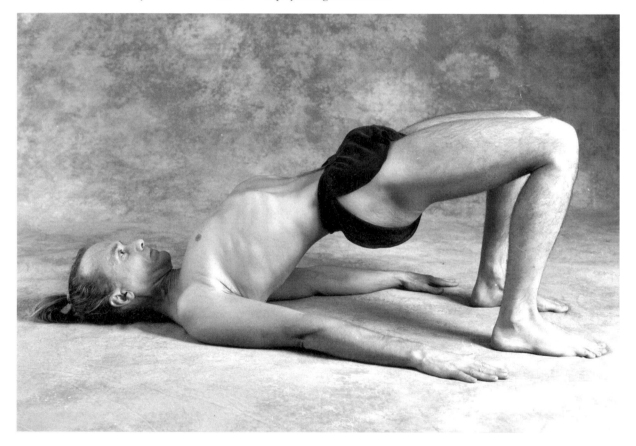

SUMMARY

Lying on the back with the feet tucked in by the buttocks, while maintaining *Uddiyana* and *Mulabandha*, alternately raise the trunk from the floor as you inhale, lowering again as you exhale. Keep hands and feet pressing down firmly throughout, with the core of the body soft. ✪5

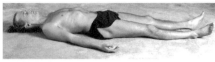

1 Lie in *Savasana*.

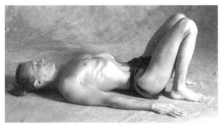

2 **Exhaling**, draw your heels in towards your buttocks, keeping your feet parallel, heels in line with the buttock bones.

3 **Inhaling**, broaden your ribcrest and suck your solar plexus in and up so your chest becomes active, broad and full, your abdomen passive, long and empty (*Uddiyanabandha*), and flatten your pubic abdomen, sucking your perineum in, with your anus soft (*Mulabandha*).

4 **Exhaling**, press the foundation of your feet, hands and shoulders down into the floor, while maintaining *Uddiyana* and *Mulabandha*.

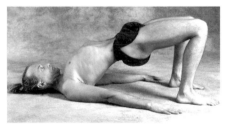

5 **Inhaling**, and maintaining an active foundation, *Uddiyana* and *Mulabandha*, raise your buttocks and spine slowly off the floor in time with your **inhalation**.

6 **Exhaling**, while maintaining an active foundation, *Uddiyana* and *Mulabandha*, lower your spine and then buttocks to the floor in time with your **exhalation**.

7 Continue to alternate between raising your body as you **inhale**, lowering as you **exhale** until your body movement is exactly synchronized with your breathing. Keep hands and feet pressing down firmly throughout, with the core of the body soft.

Once synchronicity has been established, you may stay a while in the upwards position, breathing freely with the *bandhas*. Release to the floor on an **exhalation**.

93

No. 5 Suptaikapadaparivrttasana

Supine Twist

This pose brings a gentle twist to the spine and back muscles, while softening them. Counter-pose to *Bhujadhanurasana* and all backbends, and preparation for sitting twist and backward-bending poses. It clearly teaches the role of opposition in the relationship between the bent knee and its shoulder.

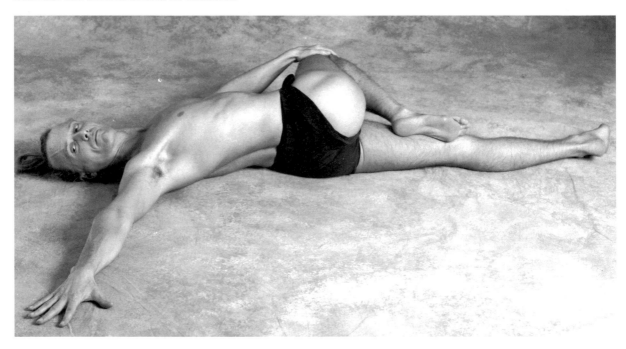

SUMMARY

Lying on the back, bend one leg placing the foot by the other knee and turn the spine and raised knee over towards the straight leg, twisting the spine.

Increase the twist with the hand on the bent knee, while looking the other way.

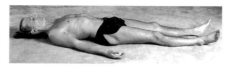

1 Lie in *Savasana*.

2 **Inhaling**, broaden your ribcrest and suck your solar plexus in and up so your chest becomes active, broad and full, your abdomen passive, long and empty (*Uddiyanabandha*), and flatten your pubic abdomen, sucking your perineum in, with your anus soft (*Mulabandha*).

3 **Exhaling**, bend your right leg and place your foot flat on the floor so that it touches the inside of your left knee.

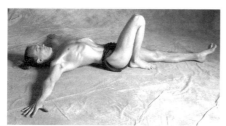

4 **Inhaling**, extend your arms out from your shoulders, palms down, so they are perpendicular to your spine.

5 **Exhaling**, raise your left hip slightly off the floor and take your right knee across the line of your body towards the floor to your left, at the same time tucking your left hip under and back.

6 **Inhaling**, clarify the *bandhas* and place your left hand gently on your right knee as you simultaneously extend your right arm out of your armpit, pressing your right shoulder down into the floor and looking towards your hand.

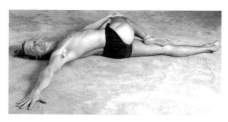

7 **Exhaling**, gently apply the weight of your left arm to your right knee so that your knee comes towards the floor. Do not allow your right shoulder to lift or you will lose the spinal twist.

After a while, release and repeat on the other side.

95

No. 6 Tadasana

Mountain Pose

This is the fundamental standing pose used for centring before and after other standing poses. It clearly reveals the current state of our alignment and imbalances. It can be held for as long as you like. It centres body, energy and mind, and awakens somatic intelligence, especially in the feet, ankles and legs. It is one of the *Suryanamaskar* postures.

SUMMARY

Stand upright, feet together, activating the *bandhas*; energize the legs, feet, arms and hands. Look straight ahead keeping the core of the body soft, with rhythmic, *Ujjayi* breathing. **7**

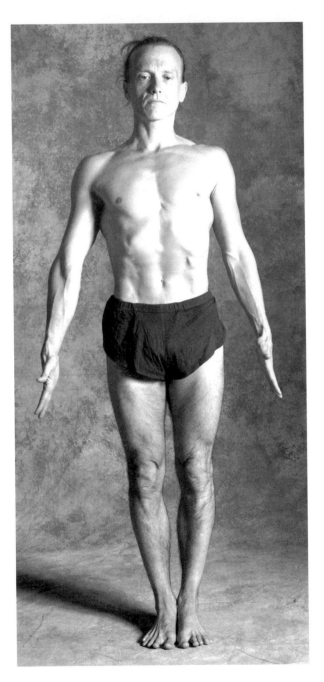

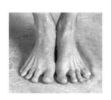

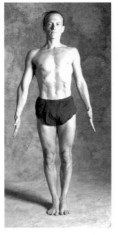

1 Stand upright with your feet together, touching at the inner heel and ball of the big toe, if possible. If not, keep your feet parallel to each other as close together as possible.

2 Spread your body weight evenly across both feet, so the heels and balls of your feet and the inner and outer edges of your feet bear the same weight. Maintain a strong, clear contact between the inner ankles, so they do not roll apart or forwards. Feel the four corners of each foot – balls of the big and little toes and the inner and outer heels – pressing down with arches lifting.

3 **Exhaling**, suck your thigh muscles into your bones so that the backs of your knees open evenly and your legs and kneecaps are centred. Your kneecaps will automatically engage.

4 **Inhaling**, lift your armpits away from your hipbones, broaden your ribcrest, and suck your solar plexus in and up so your chest becomes active, broad and full, your abdomen passive, long and empty (*Uddiyanabandha*) and, keeping your pelvic floor soft, gently lift your hipbones and engage your pubic abdomen so that it flattens and broadens as your sacrum and perineum are lifted in and up, with your anus soft (*Mulabandha*).

97

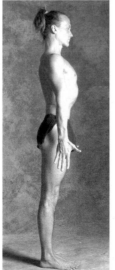

5 **Exhaling**, lengthen your neck out of your shoulders, relaxing your shoulders away from your ears, while spiralling your arms out of your armpits so that they lengthen and energize with your biceps rolling out, your wrists facing the sides of your thighs.

Hold the charge in your feet, legs, abdomen, chest, arms and hands, while looking straight ahead, core of your body soft, with smooth rhythmic *Ujjayi* breathing, till ready to release on an **exhalation**. **7**

No. 7 Urdhvahastasana

Raised Arms Pose

This pose is a continuation of *Tadasana*. It permits complete opening of your ribcage, stimulating inhalation. It can be used alongside *Tadasana* in between standing poses to re-establish breath/body synchronization. **It can be combined dynamically with *Tadasana* to develop exact breath/body synchronization.** It clarifies the action of *Uddiyanabandha*, opening the chest. It teaches the relationship between the movement of your arms and your chest and abdomen, and therefore the *bandhas*. It is one of the *Suryanamaskar* postures.

SUMMARY

Stand upright looking along the arms raised alongside the ears, palms facing each other or touching. Keep the feet together, activating the *bandhas*, energize the legs and arms, keeping the core of the body soft, with rhythmic, *Ujjayi* breathing.

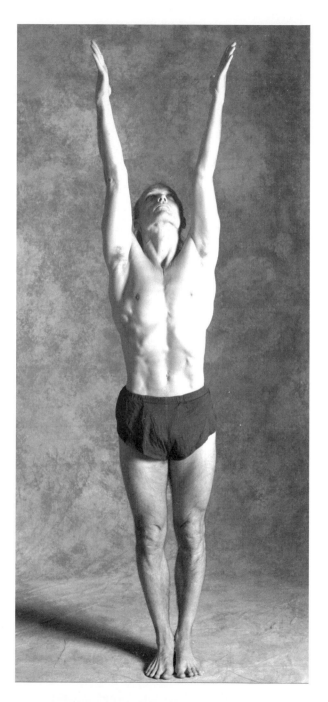

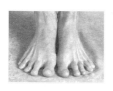

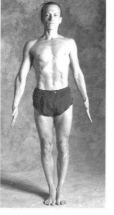

1. Stand upright with your feet together, touching at the inner heel and ball of your big toe, if possible. If not, keep your feet parallel to each other as close together as possible.

2. Spread your body weight evenly across both feet, so the heels and balls of your feet and the inner and outer edges of your feet bear the same weight. Maintain a strong, clear contact between your inner ankles, so they do not roll apart or forwards. Feel the four corners of each foot – balls of the big and little toes and the inner and outer heels – pressing down with arches lifting.

3. **Exhaling**, suck your thigh muscles into your bones so that the backs of your knees open evenly and your legs and kneecaps are centred. Your kneecaps will automatically engage.

4. **Inhaling**, lift your armpits away from your hipbones, broaden your ribcrest, and suck your solar plexus in and up so your chest becomes active, broad and full, your abdomen passive, long and empty (*Uddiyanabandha*) and, keeping your pelvic floor soft, gently lift your hipbones and engage your pubic abdomen so that it flattens and broadens as your sacrum and perineum are lifted in and up, with your anus soft (*Mulabandha*).

5. **Exhaling**, lengthen your neck out of your shoulders, relaxing them away from your ears, while spiralling your arms out of your armpits so that they lengthen and energize with the biceps rolling out, your wrists facing the sides of your thighs.

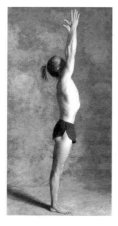

6. **Inhaling**, raise your arms up, maintaining their inner dynamic, alongside your ears, bringing your head up to gaze upwards.

Hold while looking at your palms, maintaining the *bandhas* with the core of your body soft, breath smooth and rhythmic, holding the charge in your arms and legs until ready to release on an exhalation, lowering your arms and your head with the breath.

If combined dynamically with *Tadasana*: **exhale** *Tadasana*, **inhale** *Urdhvahastasana*.

99

No. 8 Utktasana

Chair Pose

This is a dynamic, powerful pose that brings on heat rapidly. It resembles the position we take sitting on a chair. It develops strength in the front thighs and rests the hamstrings. **It can be combined dynamically with *Tadasana* or *Ardhuttanasana* to develop exact breath/body synchronization.** It teaches the importance of utilizing the ankle bone to permit balance in the legs. It is one of the *Suryanamaskar* postures.

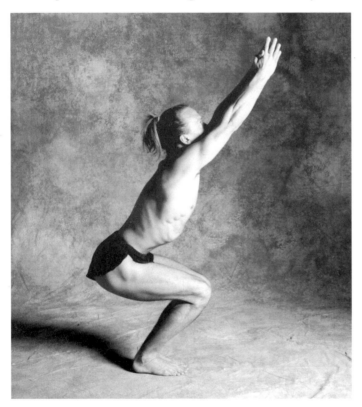

SUMMARY

Standing upright with the feet together, bend the legs, keeping the feet alive, till the thighs are parallel to the floor – while at the same time raising the arms alongside the ears, palms touching.

Maintain the *bandhas* with the abdomen long, hollow and empty, the chest broad and full, keeping the core of the body soft, with rhythmic, *Ujjayi* breathing.

10 **16**

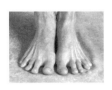

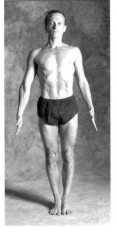

1   Stand upright with your feet together, touching at the inner heel and ball of your big toe, if possible. If not, keep your feet parallel to each other as close together as possible.

2   Spread your body weight evenly across both feet, so the heels and balls of your feet and the inner and outer edges of your feet bear the same weight. Maintain a strong, clear contact between your inner ankles, so they do not roll apart or forwards. Feel the four corners of each foot – balls of the big and little toes and the inner and outer heels – pressing down with arches lifting.

3   **Inhaling**, broaden your ribcrest and lift your arms up alongside your ears palms together and look at your palms, while sucking your solar plexus in and up so your chest becomes active, broad and full, your abdomen passive, long and empty (*Uddiyanabandha*), and keeping your pelvic floor soft gently lift your hipbones and engage your pubic abdomen so that it flattens and broadens as your sacrum is lifted in and up (*Mulabandha*).

101

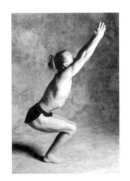

4   **Exhaling**, bend your legs, keeping your ankles together until your thighs are as close to parallel to the floor as possible.

Maintain with ankles stable, feet alive, *bandhas* engaged, core of your body soft until you are ready to release to *Tadasana* on an **exhalation**.

After a while steps **3** and **4** can be combined into a single movement on **inhaling**.

If combined dynamically with *Tadasana*: **inhale** *Utktasana*, **exhale** *Tadasana*. 10 16

No. 9 Ardhuttanasana

Gazing Pose

This pose is a preparation for the forward bend *Uttanasana*. It helps to ensure the spine is long before coming in to the legs. **It can be combined dynamically with *Uttanasana* to develop exact breath/body synchronization.** It lengthens the spine out of the pivoted pelvis, stimulates inhalation and clarifies the action of the feet and legs. It is one of the *Suryanamaskar* postures.

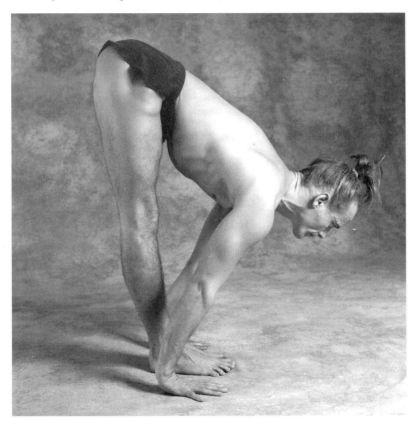

SUMMARY
With the pelvis pivoted over the tops of the thighs, hands on the floor or shins, feet alive, legs strong and straight, maintain the *bandhas* and lengthen the spine forwards and upwards while looking forwards. Keep the core of the body soft, with rhythmic, *Ujjayi* breathing.

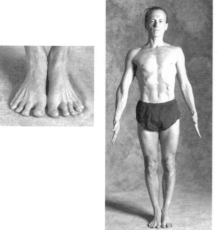

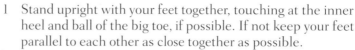

1   Stand upright with your feet together, touching at the inner heel and ball of the big toe, if possible. If not keep your feet parallel to each other as close together as possible.

2   Spread your body weight evenly across both feet, so the heels and balls of your feet and the inner and outer edges of your feet bear the same weight. Maintain a strong, clear contact between your inner ankles, so they do not roll apart or forwards. Feel the four corners of each foot – balls of the big and little toes and the inner and outer heels – pressing down with arches lifting.

3   **Exhaling**, suck your thigh muscles into your bones so that the backs of your knees open evenly and your legs and kneecaps are centred. Your kneecaps will automatically engage.

4   **Inhaling**, lift your armpits away from your hipbones, broaden your ribcrest, and suck your solar plexus in and up so your chest becomes active, broad and full, your abdomen passive, long and empty (*Uddiyanabandha*) and, keeping your pelvic floor soft, gently lift your hipbones and engage your pubic abdomen so that it flattens and broadens as your sacrum and perineum are lifted in and up, with your anus soft (*Mulabandha*).

5   **Exhaling**, keeping feet alive, legs straight and strong, pivot your pelvis over the top of your thighs bringing your palms to the floor just outside each foot, or onto your shins.

6   **Inhaling**, lift your head to gaze forward and, clarifying the *bandhas*, lengthen your spine and lift and open your chest.

103

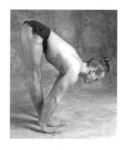

Hold with your chest broad and full, your abdomen long, hollow and empty, core of your body soft, feet alive, legs strong, spine and chest lifting. When ready to release, **inhale** into *Utktasana* by bending your legs and raising your arms, palms together alongside your ears.

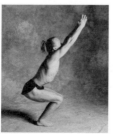

Exhaling, straighten your legs, lowering your arms into *Tadasana*.

If using dynamically with *Uttanasana*: **inhale** *Ardhuttanasana*, **exhale** *Uttanasana*.

If using dynamically with *Utktasana*: **inhale** *Ardhuttanasana*, **exhale** *Utktasana*.

No. 10 Uttanasana

Intense Stretch Pose

This pose is a demanding forward extension. **It can be combined dynamically with *Tadasana* or *Ardhuttanasana* to develop exact breath/body synchronization.** It releases the spine and pelvis, and awakens the legs and ankles, develops balance, promotes internalization and challenges *Uddiyanabandha*. It teaches the crucial role of the legs in forward extensions and the importance of the ankles to that role. Preparation for *Sirsasana*. It is one of the *Suryanamaskar* postures.

SUMMARY

With the pelvis pivoted over the tops of the thighs, feet alive, legs strong and straight, maintain the *bandhas* with the abdomen long, hollow and empty, the chest broad and full, and lengthen the spine down the legs. Keep the core of the body soft, with rhythmic, *Ujjayi* breathing. **12** **8**

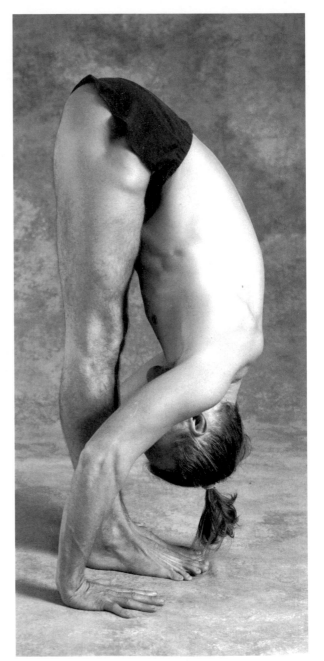

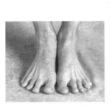

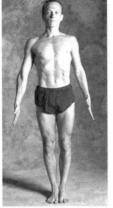

1 Stand upright with your feet together, touching at the inner heel and ball of the big toe, if possible. If not, keep your feet parallel to each other as close together as possible.

2 Spread your body weight evenly across both feet, so the heels and balls of your feet and the inner and outer edges of your feet bear the same weight. Maintain a strong, clear contact between your inner ankles, so they do not roll apart or forwards. Feel the four corners of each foot – balls of the big and little toes and the inner and outer heels – pressing down with arches lifting.

3 **Exhaling**, suck your thigh muscles into your bones so that the backs of your knees open evenly and your legs and kneecaps are centred. Your kneecaps will automatically engage.

4 **Inhaling**, lift your armpits away from your hipbones, broaden your ribcrest and suck your solar plexus in and up so your chest becomes active, broad and full, your abdomen passive, long and empty (*Uddiyanabandha*) and, keeping your pelvic floor soft, gently lift your hipbones and engage your pubic abdomen so that it flattens and broadens as your sacrum and perineum are lifted in and up with your anus soft (*Mulabandha*).

105

5 **Exhaling**, keeping feet alive, legs straight and strong, pivot your pelvis over the top of your thighs, bringing your palms to the floor just outside each foot, or onto the shinbones.

6 **Inhaling**, lift your head to gaze forward and, clarifying the *bandhas*, lengthen your spine and lift and open your chest.

7 **Exhaling**, bend your arms and lengthen your spine down the legs, taking your chin towards your feet.

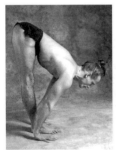

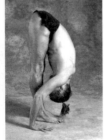

Hold with chest broad and full, your abdomen long, hollow and empty, feet alive, legs strong, spine and chest lifting. To release, **inhale** into *Utktasana* by bending your legs and raising your arms, palms together alongside your ears then, exhaling, straighten your legs, lowering your arms into *Tadasana*.

If using dynamically with *Ardhuttanasana*: **inhale** *Ardhuttanasana*, **exhale** *Uttanasana*.

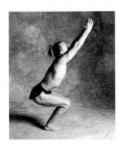

If using dynamically with *Utktasana*: **inhale** *Utktasana*, **exhale** *Uttanasana*. **12** **8**

No. 11 Ardhachaturangadandasana

Half Crocodile

This pose resembles a crocodile. It awakens the legs and teaches the correct use of the hands when bearing weight. Keep the ribcage on the floor. Preparation for *Chaturangadandasana*. It is one of the *Sukhasuryanamaskar* postures.

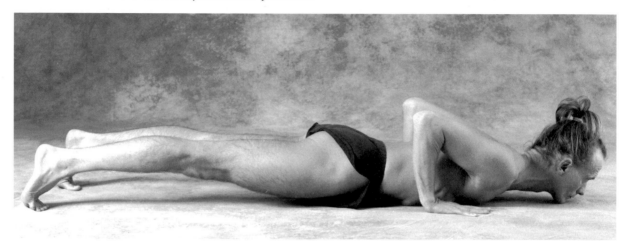

SUMMARY

From a face-down position, suck the leg muscles into the bones so that the legs straighten and lift from the floor. At the same time, engage the hands and lift the pelvis and navel off the floor. Keep the ribcage on the floor. Throughout maintain the action of the *bandhas*, keeping the core of the body soft, with rhythmic, *Ujjayi* breathing. ✸15 ✸13

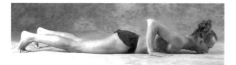

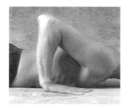

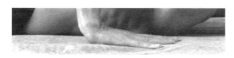

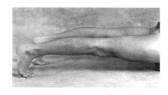

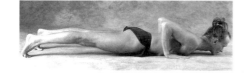

1   Lie face down on the floor, legs straight with toes tucked in towards your pelvis, feet hip-width apart, head centred, hands behind your armpits close in by your side chest so that your forearms are perpendicular, with your wrists directly under your elbows.

2   **Inhaling**, broaden your ribcrest and suck your solar plexus in and up so your chest becomes active, broad and full, your abdomen passive, long and empty (*Uddiyanabandha*), and flatten your pubic abdomen, sucking your perineum and sacrum in with your anus soft (*Mulabandha*).

3   **Exhaling**, engage your hands with the floor so that they make full contact, palms broad, fingers long, index fingerbase pressing down.

4   **Inhaling**, clarify the *bandhas* and soften the core of your body.

5   **Exhaling**, fully engage your legs by sucking the muscles into the bone so that the backs of your knees open and the fronts of your thighs and shins lift off the floor, and lift your hips and navel just off the floor.

Keep your ribcage on the floor.

Hold with your abdomen and hips parallel to the floor while maintaining the action of the *bandhas*, hands and legs. Keep the core of your body soft, with smooth, rhythmic *Ujjayi* breathing. Release as you **inhale**, keeping the action of the *bandhas*, hands and legs until you are fully relaxed onto the floor. ✹ ✹

107

No. 12 Chaturangadandasana

The Crocodile

This pose requires and develops balanced upper body strength. The key is the position and use of the hands, and the utilization of the full power of the legs, so that an even distribution of weight and even utilization of muscles results. It awakens the legs and develops stability and strength in the limbs and in the trunk. Preparation for *Urdhvamukhasvanasana*. It is one of the *Suryanamaskar* postures.

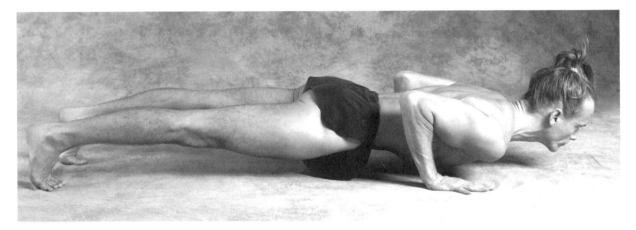

SUMMARY

From a face-down position, suck the leg muscles into the bones so that the legs straighten and lift from the floor. At the same time, engage the hands and lift the upper body fractionally off the floor.

Keep the whole body parallel to the floor, supported by the hands and feet. Throughout maintain the action of the *bandhas*, keeping the core of the body soft, with rhythmic, *Ujjayi* breathing. **15**

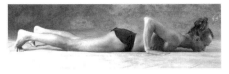

1 Lie face down on the floor, legs straight with toes tucked in towards your pelvis, feet hip-width apart, head centred, hands behind your armpits close in by your side chest so that your forearms are perpendicular, with your wrists directly under your elbows.

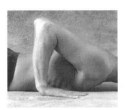

2 **Inhaling**, broaden your ribcrest and suck your solar plexus in and up so your chest becomes active, broad and full, your abdomen passive, long and empty (*Uddiyanabandha*), and flatten your pubic abdomen, sucking your perineum and sacrum in with your anus soft (*Mulabandha*).

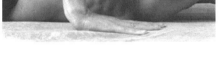

3 **Exhaling**, engage your hands with the floor so that they make full contact, palms broad, fingers long, index fingerbase pressing down.

4 **Inhaling**, clarify the *bandhas* and soften the core of your body.

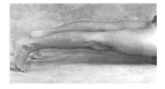

5 **Exhaling**, fully engage your legs by sucking the muscles into the bone, so that the backs of your knees open, and the fronts of your thighs and shins lift off the floor, while at the same time lifting your pelvis, abdomen and ribcage just off the floor.

109

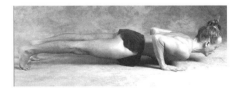

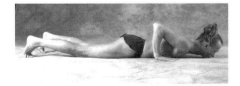

Hold your whole body parallel to the floor, while maintaining the action of the *bandhas*, hands and legs, keeping the core of your body soft, with smooth, rhythmic *Ujjayi* breathing. Release as you **exhale**, keeping the action of the *bandhas*, hands and legs until you are fully relaxed onto the floor. **15**

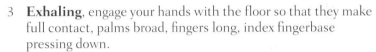

No. 13 Ardhurdhvamukhasvanasana

Half Upward Dog

This pose resembles a dog stretching its upper back gently. It is an easy, preparatory version of the full pose shown next. It strengthens the legs and teaches the correct use of the hands. It opens the intervertebral spaces in the top spine; opens the chest; releases tension in the shoulders; and mobilizes the neck. Preparation for *Urdhvamukhasvanasana* and backbends. It is one of the *Sukhasuryanamaskar* postures.

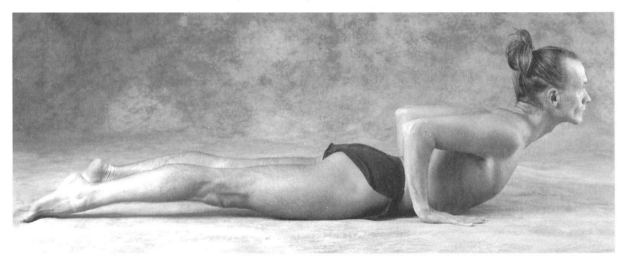

110

SUMMARY

From a face-down position, keeping the legs straight and strong, tops of the feet on the floor hip-width apart and long, use the hands behind the armpits to raise the chest and head upwards off the floor, while maintaining the action of the *bandhas*, hands and legs, keeping the core of the body soft, with rhythmic, *Ujjayi* breathing. **64** **14**

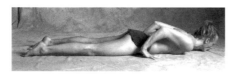

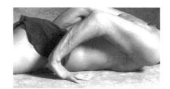

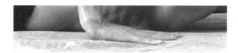

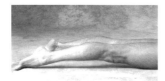

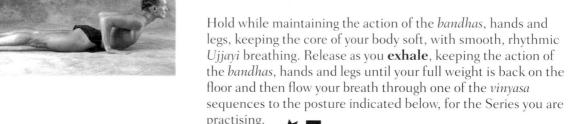

1 Lie face down on the floor, legs straight with toes stretched back away from the body, front ankle long, feet hip-width apart. Keep your head centred, hands near your hips, fingers pointing forwards.

2 **Inhaling**, broaden your ribcrest and suck your solar plexus in and up so your chest becomes active, broad and full, your abdomen passive, long and empty (*Uddiyanabandha*), and flatten your pubic abdomen, sucking your perineum and sacrum in with your anus soft (*Mulabandha*).

3 **Exhaling**, engage your hands with the floor so that they make full contact, palms broad, fingers long, index fingerbase pressing down.

4 **Inhaling**, clarify the *bandhas* and soften the core of your body.

5 **Exhaling**, fully engage your legs by sucking the muscles into the bone so that the backs of your knees open, keeping the front of your legs in contact with and pushing down into the floor.

6 **Inhaling**, fully engage your hands and, pressing from the index fingerbase, raise your chin and chest from the floor, but keep your ribcrest down in contact with the floor.

7 **Exhaling**, clarify the action of the *bandhas*, hands and legs.

8 **Inhaling**, lift your head up and look straight ahead.

Hold while maintaining the action of the *bandhas*, hands and legs, keeping the core of your body soft, with smooth, rhythmic *Ujjayi* breathing. Release as you **exhale**, keeping the action of the *bandhas*, hands and legs until your full weight is back on the floor and then flow your breath through one of the *vinyasa* sequences to the posture indicated below, for the Series you are practising. ✹64 ■14

111

No. 14 Urdhvamukhasvanasana

Upwards Dog Pose

This pose is a powerful, demanding backbend. The legs must be kept powerful, without tension in the buttocks or pelvic floor, to protect the lumbar spine from pinching. It opens the chest, mobilizes the spine and develops the arms and legs. Counterbalance to forward extensions. It teaches the role of the legs and *bandhas* in supporting the lumbar spine during backbends. It is one of the *Suryanamaskar* postures.

112

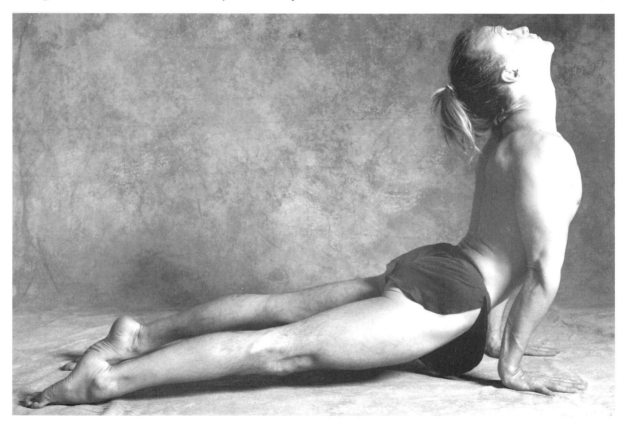

SUMMARY
From a face-down position, tops of the feet on the floor hip-width apart and long, keeping the legs straight and strong, raise them off the floor pressing the tops of the feet down and, drawing the hips forwards as they come just off the floor, use the hands to raise the chest and head upwards off the floor, while maintaining the action of the *bandhas*, hands and legs, keeping the core of the body soft, with rhythmic, *Ujjayi* breathing.

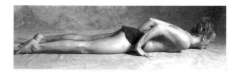

1 Lie face down on the floor, legs straight with toes stretched back away from the body, front ankle long, feet hip-width apart. Keep your head centred, hands close in by your abdomen.

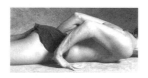

2 **Inhaling**, broaden your ribcrest and suck your solar plexus in and up so your chest becomes active, broad and full, your abdomen passive, long and empty (*Uddiyanabandha*), and flatten your pubic abdomen, sucking your perineum and sacrum in with your anus soft (*Mulabandha*).

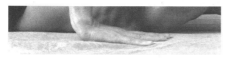

3 **Exhaling**, engage your hands with the floor so that they make full contact, palms broad, fingers long, index fingerbase pressing down.

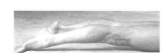

4 **Inhaling**, clarify the *bandhas* and soften the core of your body.

5 **Exhaling**, fully engage your legs by sucking the muscles into the bone so that the backs of the knees open.

113

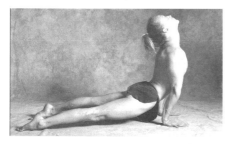

6 **Inhaling**, fully engage your hands and, pressing from the index fingerbase, arch your back and raise your chin, chest and navel from the floor, while at the same time drawing your hips forwards to your hands and lifting the fronts of your legs off the floor, while pressing the tops of your feet and your pubis down. Hold your whole body off the floor except for your hands and the tops of your feet from the toes to the front ankle, while maintaining the action of the *bandhas*, hands and legs, keeping the core of the body soft, with smooth, rhythmic *Ujjayi* breathing. Release as you **exhale**, keeping the action of the *bandhas*, hands and legs until your full weight is back on the floor.

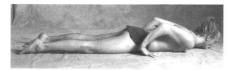

In *Suryanamaskar*, **exhale** to *Adhomukhasvanasana* (**15**). In the Foundation series follow the breath through *Svanavinyasa* to *Ardhasarvangasana* (**65**).

Urdhvamukhasvanasana can also be entered from *Chaturangadandasana*. **Exhale** into *Chaturangadandasana* (**12**) and then **inhale** and drag the hips forwards as you lift up into *Urdhvamukhasvanasana*.

65

No. 15 Adhomukhasvanasana

Downward Dog

This pose resembles a dog stretching its whole body, and is an important pose for awakening the limbs and, when mastered, for resting in. It relieves the heart, awakens the whole body and releases tension from the trunk. Preparation for *Sirsasana*. It teaches the interrelationship of each part to every other and to the whole, and facilitates the awakening of somatic intelligence. It is one of the *Suryanamaskar* postures.

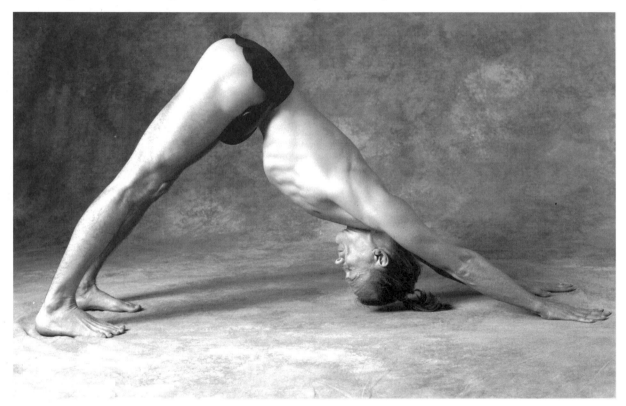

SUMMARY

From a lying position with feet hip-width apart, push the trunk off the floor straightening the arms and legs (or, from all fours, straighten the legs) so the hips rise up while the head goes back and stays down. Maintain the *bandhas* with the abdomen long, hollow and empty, the chest broad and full, keep the spirallic charge of arms and legs, with the hands and feet alive and even. Keep the neck relaxed, core of the body soft with smooth, rhythmic *Ujjayi* breathing. *Sukhasuryanamaskar*

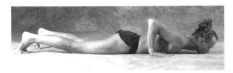

1 Lie face down on the floor, legs straight with toes tucked in towards the pelvis, feet hip-width apart, head centred, hands behind your armpits close in by your side chest so that your forearms are perpendicular with your wrists directly under your elbows.

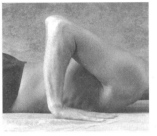

2 **Exhaling**, engage your hands with the floor so that they make full contact, palms broad, fingers long, index fingerbase pressing down.

3 **Inhaling**, broaden your ribcrest and suck your solar plexus in and up so your chest becomes active, broad and full, your abdomen passive, long and empty (*Uddiyanabandha*), and flatten your pubic abdomen, sucking your perineum and sacrum in with your anus soft (*Mulabandha*).

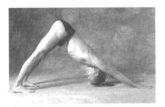

4 **Exhaling**, push from your index fingerbase and straighten your legs, sucking your thigh muscles in, so your hips rise up, and lower your head to look back through your legs, neck completely relaxed.

115

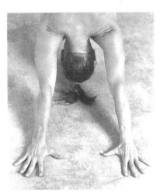

5 **Inhaling**, clarify the *bandhas* and the spirallic action of your arms and legs. Lift your upper shoulders out and up, while pressing your inner wrist down to spiral your arms. Similarly, hit your inner ankle back, while hitting your outer hip back, with your kneecaps centred.

Hold as long as you wish, keeping your neck relaxed with a strong lifting charge in your arms and legs, with smooth, rhythmic *Ujjayi* breathing, core of your body soft, and **inhale** to release back to the floor. ✱ *Sukhasuryanamaskar*

No. 16 Trikonasana

Triangle Pose

This simple pose makes the whole body alive and strong. It awakens the feet and legs. It teaches the relationship between the use of the legs and the quality of the pelvic floor. Preparation for asymmetrical standing poses. Counter-pose for bent leg standing poses.

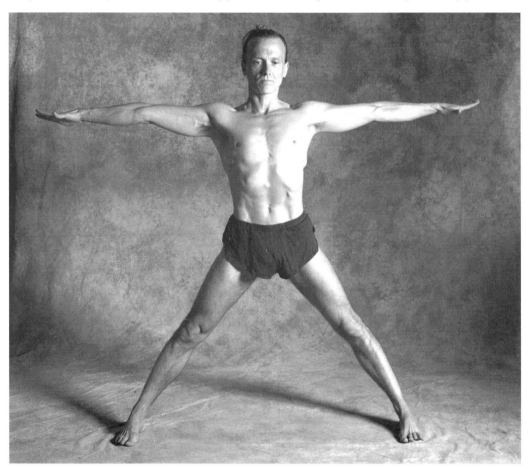

SUMMARY

With the feet wide apart and arches lifting with the four corners pressing down equally, stand strong and stable with weight even on the feet, legs straight and bracing apart, hands alive with arms parallel to the floor, *bandhas* engaged, core of the body soft and enjoying rhythmic, effortless *Ujjayi* breathing. **22** **17**

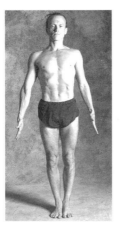

1 Start in *Tadasana*.

As you **inhale**, turn to the right and step your feet wide apart, hands on hips.

2 **Exhaling**, spread your body weight evenly across both feet, so the heels and balls of your feet and the inner and outer edges of your feet bear the same weight. Maintain a strong, clear contact between your inner ankles, so they do not roll apart or forwards. Feel the four corners of each foot – balls of the big and little toes and the inner and outer heels – pressing down with arches lifting. If you need more time, breathe freely.

3 **Inhaling**, suck your thigh muscles into your bones so that the backs of your knees open evenly and your legs and kneecaps are centred. Your kneecaps will automatically engage.

4 **Exhaling** brace the inner planes of your legs apart creating space across your pelvic floor, and feeling your outer knees and hips gripping.

117

5 **Inhaling**, keeping your pelvic floor soft, gently lift your hipbones while engaging your pubic abdomen so that it flattens and broadens as your sacrum is lifted in and up (*Mulabandha*) and broaden your ribcrest, sucking your solar plexus in and up so your chest becomes active, broad and full, your abdomen passive, long and empty (*Uddiyanabandha*), and lifting your armpits away from your hipbones.

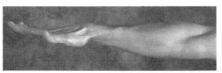

6 **Exhaling**, lengthen your neck out of your shoulders, relaxing them away from your ears.

7 **Inhaling**, spiral your arms out of your armpits parallel to the floor so that they lengthen and energize with your biceps up rolling out, the wrists keeping the palms flat.

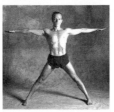

Hold the charge in legs, arms, feet, hands, abdomen and chest with smooth rhythmic *Ujjayi* breathing, core of the body soft, while looking straight till ready to release back to *Tadasana* on an **exhalation**. 22 17

No. 17 Utthitatrikonasana

Extended Triangle Pose

This is the most important posture for awakening somatic intelligence throughout the whole body. Simple in its shape, it is complex in its subtlety. It provides a firm, indispensable foundation for more strenuous postures, strengthens the legs, develops the feet, releases the pelvis, opens the chest, releases the neck. Preparation for *Parsvakonasana* and *Parsvavirabhadrasana*. It teaches the interrelationship of each part to every other and to the whole.

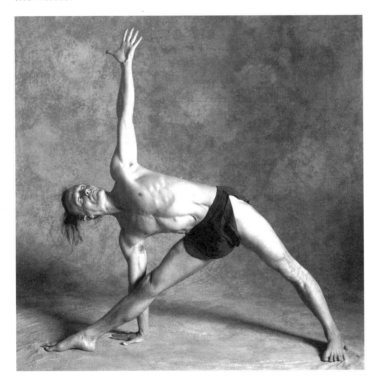

SUMMARY

Feet wide apart, turn the front foot out 90 degrees, the back foot in 15/25 degrees, arches lifting with the four corners pressing down equally and legs straight and strong. Tuck in the front hip as you extend the trunk along the line of the front leg, then, without dropping the armpit, take that hand to the floor, with spine parallel to the floor. Stretch the top arm up with the head turned to look at it. Maintain the *bandhas* with the abdomen long, hollow and empty, the chest broad and full and the charge in hands, feet, arms and legs, with smooth, rhythmic *Ujjayi* breathing. **18**

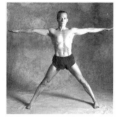

1 Start in *Tadasana*. As you **inhale**, turn to the right and step your feet wide apart, with your arms parallel to the floor. You are now in *Trikonasana*.

2 **Exhaling**, turn your right foot out 90 degrees, and your left foot 15/25 degrees in without dropping your knee in. Line up the heel of your right foot with the ankle of your left foot.

3 **Inhaling**, broaden your ribcrest and suck your solar plexus in and up so your chest becomes active, broad and full, your abdomen passive, long and empty (*Uddiyanabandha*), and flatten your pubic abdomen, sucking your perineum and sacrum in with your anus soft (*Mulabandha*), keeping a strong charge in arms and legs.

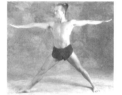

4 **Exhaling**, keep both hips on the plane defined by your front heel and the arch of your back foot by hitting the outer edge of your left knee backwards and rolling your left hip backwards and tucking your right buttock in.

119

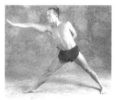

5 **Inhaling**, tuck your right hip in by rotating the pubic bone around its centre, so your right hip drops as the left lifts, and extend your right arm forwards as far as possible, so that the whole of the right side of your trunk lengthens out of the rotating pelvis. Steps **4** and **5** combined will bring your right armpit down towards the level of your right hip, without any bending at the waist. At the same time take your left arm behind your waist.

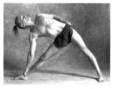

6 **Exhaling**, lengthen your right arm and take your right hand down to the floor, or to your ankle or shin.

7 **Inhaling**, lengthen your left arm vertically out of your armpit and, turning your whole trunk upwards, look at your left hand.

Hold the charge in legs, arms, feet, hands, abdomen and chest with smooth rhythmic *Ujjayi* breathing, core of your body soft, until ready to release, then, **inhaling**, lift back up to *Trikonasana* again.

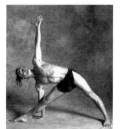

Repeat steps **2 to 8** to the left. Then, exhaling, turn and step back to *Tadasana*.

18

No. 18 Parivrttatrikonasana

Revolving Triangle Pose

This pose gives an easy twist to the spine and back muscles. The legs must be kept strong, the pelvis parallel to the floor. It strengthens the legs, opens the pelvis and releases the spine and neck. Preparation and compensation for backwards bending, and *Virabhadrasana*. It teaches the relationship between feet, legs, pelvis and spine.

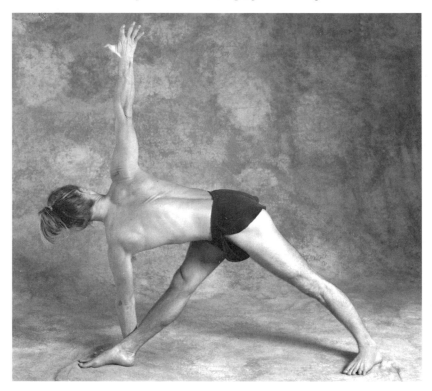

SUMMARY

With the feet wide apart turn the front foot out 90 degrees, the back foot 75 degrees, and bring the back hip in line with the front, so the whole trunk is facing directly forwards. Keep the arches of the feet lifting with the four corners pressing down equally. Keeping the legs strong, pivot the pelvis, turn the trunk and rotate the spine so the back hand comes down outside the front foot, with the front arm extending upwards. Look at the top hand. Maintain the *bandhas* with the abdomen long, hollow and empty, the chest broad and full, with smooth rhythmic *Ujjayi* breathing, core of the body soft. Keep strong legs and arms, hands and feet alive.

20

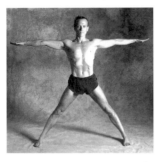

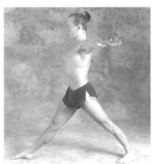

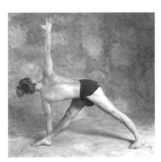

1 Start in *Tadasana*. As you **inhale**, turn to the right and step your feet wide apart, with your arms parallel to the floor. You are now in *Trikonasana*.

2 **Exhaling**, turn your right foot out 90 degrees, and your left foot in 75 degrees, turning the whole leg with it. Line up the heel of your right foot with the ankle of your left foot. Turn your trunk with your legs to bring your left hip forward in line with your right, keeping your arms outstretched parallel to the floor.

3 **Inhaling**, broaden your ribcrest and suck your solar plexus in and up so your chest becomes active, broad and full, your abdomen passive, long and empty (*Uddiyanabandha*), and flatten your pubic abdomen, sucking your perineum and sacrum in with your anus soft (*Mulabandha*), keeping a strong charge in arms and legs.

4 **Exhaling**, rotate your spine keeping it long and straight as you sweep your left hand to the floor outside the right foot (or on to the shinbone), as your right arm goes vertical.

121

5 **Inhaling**, lengthen your arms and turn your head to gaze and your upstretched left hand above its shoulder, keeping the right side of your trunk long.

Hold your charge in legs, arms, feet, hands, abdomen and chest with smooth rhythmic *Ujjayi* breathing, core of your body soft, until ready to release, **inhaling** as you raise your trunk back up to *Trikonasana*.

Repeat **2 to 5** to the left. Then turn and step back to *Tadasana*. **20**

No. 19 Salambaparsvakonasana

Supported Lunge Pose

This pose gives a clear stretch to each side of the body. It opens the pelvis, lengthens the spine, frees the chest, develops the feet and legs. It gives a gentle twist to the spine. Preparation for *Parsvakonasana* and *Parsvavirabhadrasana*. It teaches how to lengthen the side trunk without bending the waist.

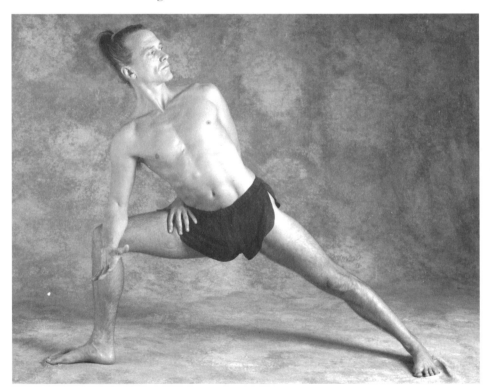

SUMMARY
Feet wide apart, turn the front foot out 90 degrees, the back foot in 15/25 degrees, and bend the front leg to a right angle, resisting with the back leg. Keep the arches of the feet lifting with the four corners pressing down equally. Extend the spine out of the pelvis over the front leg with the back arm behind the waist. Press the front elbow on the front thigh as you lengthen and turn, looking over the left shoulder. Maintain the *bandhas* with the abdomen long, hollow and empty, the chest broad and full, core of the body soft, strong legs and arms, hands and feet alive, with smooth, rhythmic *Ujjayi* breathing.

24

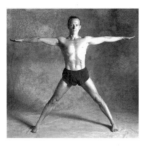

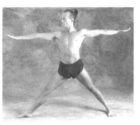

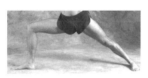

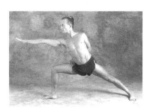

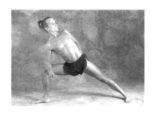

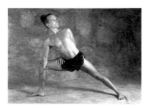

1   Start in *Tadasana*. As you **inhale**, turn to the right and step your feet wide apart, with your arms parallel to the floor. You are now in *Trikonasana*.

2   **Exhaling**, turn your right foot out 90 degrees, and your left foot in 15/25 degrees, without dropping your knee in. Line up the heel of your right foot with the ankle of your left foot.

3   **Inhaling**, broaden your ribcrest and suck your solar plexus in and up so your chest becomes active, broad and full, your abdomen passive, long and empty (*Uddiyanabandha*), and flatten your pubic abdomen, sucking your perineum and sacrum in with your anus soft (*Mulabandha*), keeping a strong charge in arms and legs.

4   **Exhaling**, sucking your thigh muscles in, hit the outer edge of your left knee backwards and roll your left hip backwards.

5   **Inhaling**, lengthen your spine and open your chest.

6   **Exhaling**, resist with your left leg by hitting inner knee out, your outer knee back, and bend your right leg until you have a right angle, knee directly above the ankle, shin bone perpendicular, thigh bone parallel to the floor.

7   **Inhaling**, with your left arm behind your waist, extend your right arm and side of the trunk forwards out of your pelvis. Keep the left hip and right buttock in line.

8   **Exhaling**, lower your right elbow on to your right thigh by your knee.

9   **Inhaling**, turn your trunk and head to look up over your left shoulder as you lengthen your spine, pressing with your right arm on your right thigh, and gripping the top of your right thigh with your left hand.

Hold the charge in legs, arms, feet, hands, abdomen and chest with smooth rhythmic *Ujjayi* breathing, core of your body soft, until ready to release by raising back up to *Trikonasana* on an **inhalation**.

Repeat to the left steps **2 to 9**, then turn and step back to *Tadasana* while **exhaling**. 24

123

No. 20 Parsvakonasana

Lunge Pose

This pose gives a deep stretch to each side of the body. Keep the pelvis aligned on the plane of the feet. It opens the pelvis, lengthens the spine, frees the chest, and develops the feet and legs. It teaches the importance of the use of the legs and pelvis in supporting the action of the spine.

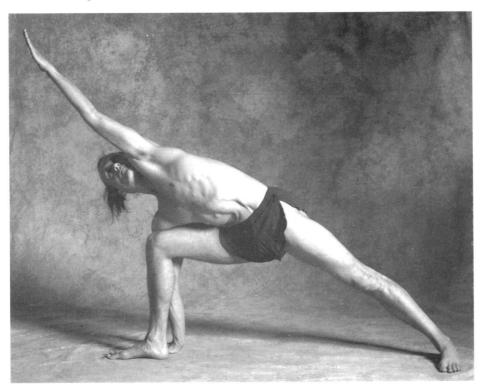

SUMMARY

Feet wide apart, turn the front foot out 90 degrees, the back foot in 15/25 degrees, and bend the front leg to a right angle, resisting with the back leg. Keep the arches of the feet lifting with the four corners pressing down equally. Extend the spine out of the pelvis along the front leg with the back arm extending forward alongside the ear, and the front hand coming to the floor outside the front knee. Press the knee into the elbow and look along the top arm. Maintain the *bandhas* with the abdomen long, hollow and empty, the chest broad and full, core of the body soft, strong legs and arms, hands and feet alive, with smooth, rhythmic *Ujjayi* breathing. **21**

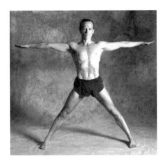

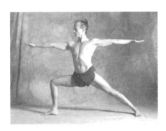

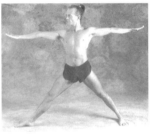

1 Start in *Tadasana*. As you **inhale**, turn to the right and step your feet wide apart, with your arms parallel to the floor. You are now in *Trikonasana*.
2 **Exhaling**, turn your right foot out 90 degrees, and your left foot in 15/25 degrees without dropping your knee in. Line up the heel of your right foot with the ankle of your left foot.
3 **Inhaling**, broaden your ribcrest and suck your solar plexus in and up so your chest becomes active, broad and full, your abdomen passive, long and empty (*Uddiyanabandha*), and flatten your pubic abdomen, sucking your perineum and sacrum in with your anus soft (*Mulabandha*), keeping a strong charge in arms and legs.
4 **Exhaling**, sucking your thigh muscles in, hit the outer edge of your left knee backwards and roll your left hip backwards.
5 **Inhaling**, lengthen your spine and open your chest.
6 **Exhaling**, resist with the left leg by hitting your inner knee out, your outer knee back, and bend your right leg until you have a right angle, knee directly above the ankle, shin bone perpendicular, thigh bone parallel to the floor.
7 **Inhaling**, with your left arm behind your waist, extend your right arm and side of the trunk forwards out of your pelvis. Keep your left hip and right buttock in line.
8 **Exhaling**, lower your right hand to the floor outside your right foot. Press your right knee hard into your right armpit and tuck your right buttock in.
9 **Inhaling**, turn your trunk and head to look up over your left shoulder as you lengthen your spine.
10 **Exhaling**, bring your left arm forward alongside your left ear and look along the arm, keeping it at the same angle from the floor as your left leg. Gently turn your spine and chest upwards.

Hold the charge in legs, arms, feet, hands, abdomen and chest with smooth, rhythmic *Ujjayi* breathing, core of your body soft, until ready to release by raising back up to *Trikonasana* on an **inhalation**.

Repeat to the left steps **2 to 10**, then turn and step back to *Tadasana* while **exhaling**. **21**

125

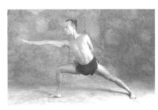

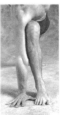
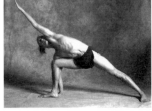

No. 21 Namaskarparvritaparsvakonasana

Revolving Lunge Pose

This pose enables accurate visual control of the alignment of the front thigh and buttock when the leg is bent to a right angle at the knee. It strengthens the legs and feet, releases the ankles, mobilizes the pelvis, releases the spine, softens the back and frees the neck. Preparation, counter-pose for backward bendings, and *Virabhadrasana*.

126

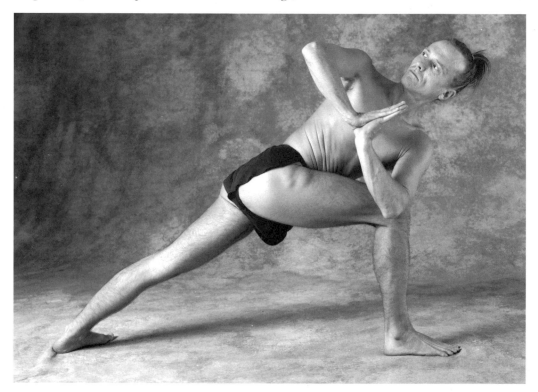

SUMMARY

With feet wide apart, turn the front foot out 90 degrees, the back foot 75 degrees and bring the back hip in line with the front. Keep the arches of the feet lifting with the four corners pressing down equally. Bend the front leg, making a right angle at the knee and, rotating the spine towards the bent leg, extend it forwards and place the bottom elbow outside the knee. Press the top palm on to the bottom with forearms straight and look past the top elbow. Maintain the *bandhas* with the abdomen long, hollow and empty, the chest broad and full, with smooth, rhythmic *Ujjayi* breathing, core of the body soft. Keep strong legs and arms, hands and feet alive. **23**

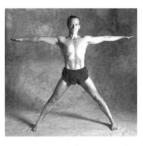

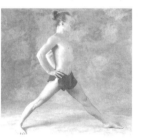

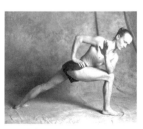

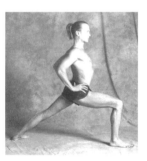

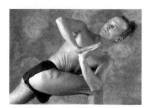

1   Start in *Tadasana*. As you **inhale**, turn to the right and step your feet wide apart, with your arms parallel to the floor. You are now in *Trikonasana*.

2   **Exhaling**, turn your right foot out 90 degrees, and your left foot in 75 degrees, turning your whole leg with it. Line up the heel of your right foot with the ankle of your left foot. Turn your trunk with your legs to bring your left hip forward in line with your right, bringing your hands to your hips.

3   **Inhaling**, broaden your ribcrest and suck your solar plexus in and up so your chest becomes active, broad and full, your abdomen passive, long and empty (*Uddiyanabandha*), and flatten your pubic abdomen, sucking your perineum and sacrum in with your anus soft (*Mulabandha*), keeping a strong charge in arms and legs.

4   **Exhaling**, keeping your left leg straight and strong, bend your right leg till you have a right angle at the knee, thighbone parallel, shinbone perpendicular to the floor.

5   **Inhaling**, turn and extend your trunk forward, leading with your elbow so that it reaches the outside of your right knee.

6   **Exhaling**, pressing your left elbow into your right knee while resisting with the knee, bring your palms together so that as they press into each other your two forearms make a straight line, angling upwards.

7   **Inhaling**, turn your spine to the right and look past your right elbow.

Hold maintaining the *bandhas* with legs strong until ready to release by raising back up to *Trikonasana* on an **inhalation**.

Repeat to the left steps **2 to 8**, then turn and step back to *Tadasana* while **exhaling**. **23**

127

No. 22 Urdhvapadottanasana

Gazing Pose

This pose awakens the feet and legs, while at the same time lengthening the spine, releasing the neck and clarifying the *bandhas*. It teaches the relationship between the use of the legs and the quality of the pelvic floor.

128

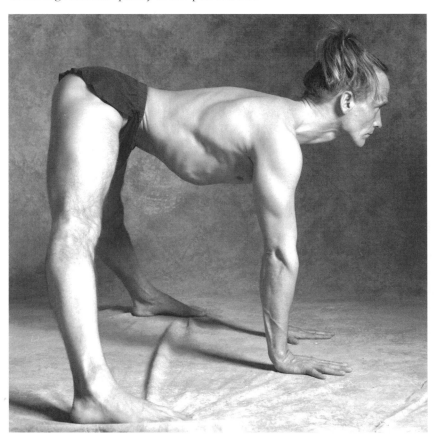

SUMMARY

With feet wide apart and parallel, legs straight and strong, pivot the pelvis, bring the hands to the floor and extend the spine out of the pelvis parallel to the floor looking straight ahead. Keep the arches of the feet lifting with the four corners pressing down equally. Maintain the *bandhas* with the abdomen long, hollow and empty, the chest broad and full, with smooth rhythmic *Ujjayi* breathing, core of the body soft. Keep the charge in legs, arms, feet and hands.

23

1 From *Tadasana* turn and spread the feet wide apart and parallel to each other.

2 **Exhaling**, spread your body weight evenly across both feet, so the heels and balls of your feet and the inner and outer edges of your feet bear the same weight. Maintain a strong, clear contact between your inner ankles, so they do not roll apart or forwards. Feel the four corners of each foot – balls of the big and little toes and the inner and outer heels – pressing down with arches lifting. If you need more time, breathe freely.

3 **Inhaling**, suck your thigh muscles into your bones so that the backs of your knees open evenly and your legs and kneecaps are centred. Your kneecaps will automatically engage.

4 **Exhaling**, brace the inner planes of your legs apart, creating space across the pelvic floor, and feeling the outer knees and hips gripping.

129

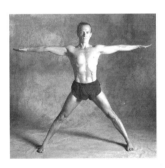

5 **Inhaling**, keeping your pelvic floor soft, gently lift your hipbones while engaging your pubic abdomen so that it flattens and broadens as your sacrum is lifted in and up (*Mulabandha*) and broaden your ribcrest, sucking your solar plexus in and up so your chest becomes active, broad and full, your abdomen passive, long and empty (*Uddiyanabandha*). Lift your armpits away from your hipbones and extend your arms out parallel to the floor.

6 **Exhaling**, pivot your pelvis and, as your spine comes down parallel to the floor, place your hands on the floor underneath your shoulders.

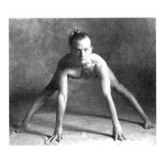

7 **Inhaling**, lift your head and look straight forwards.

Hold the charge in legs, arms, feet, hands, abdomen and chest with smooth rhythmic *Ujjayi* breathing, core of your body soft, till ready to return to *Trikonasana* on an **inhalation**, then turn and step back to *Tadasana* on an **exhalation**. **23**

No. 23 Padottanasana

Leg Stretch Pose

This pose is the easiest one for awakening the feet and legs, while at the same time challenging the *bandhas*. It is a restful pose for the trunk and the heart. It teaches the relationship between the use of the legs and the quality of the pelvic floor.

130

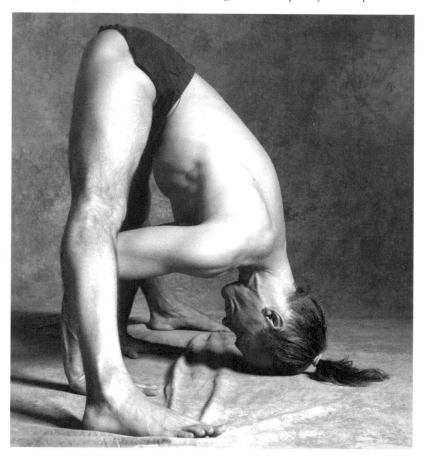

SUMMARY

With feet wide apart and legs straight and strong take, the palms to the floor under the shoulders, relaxing the neck and spine. Keep the arches of the feet lifting with the four corners pressing down equally. Maintain the *bandhas* with the abdomen long, hollow and empty, the chest broad and full. Keep the charge in legs, arms, feet and hands with smooth rhythmic *Ujjayi* breathing, core of the body soft. **19** **25**

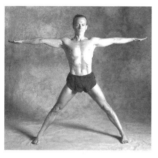

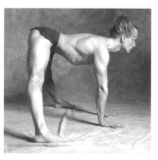

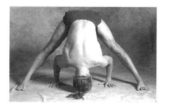

1   From *Tadasana* turn and spread your feet wide apart and parallel to each other.

2   **Exhaling**, spread your body weight evenly across both feet, so the heels and balls of your feet and the inner and outer edges of your feet bear the same weight. Maintain a strong, clear contact between your inner ankles, so they do not roll apart or forwards. Feel the four corners of each foot – balls of the big and little toes and the inner and outer heels – pressing down with arches lifting. If you need more time, breathe freely.

3   **Inhaling**, suck your thigh muscles into the bones so that the backs of your knees open evenly and your legs and kneecaps are centred. Your kneecaps will automatically engage.

4   **Exhaling**, brace the inner planes of your legs apart, creating space across your pelvic floor, and feeling the outer knees and hips gripping.

131

5   **Inhaling**, keeping your pelvic floor soft, gently lift your hipbones while engaging your pubic abdomen so that it flattens and broadens as your sacrum is lifted in and up (*Mulabandha*) and broaden your ribcrest, sucking your solar plexus in and up so your chest becomes active, broad and full, your abdomen passive, long and empty (*Uddiyanabandha*). Lift your armpits away from your hipbones, and extend your arms out parallel to the floor.

6   **Exhaling**, pivot your pelvis and take your palms to the floor.

7   **Inhaling**, lift your head and look straight forwards.

8   **Exhaling**, take your hands as far back as you can with palms flat on the floor, in line with your shoulders. Keep your forearms vertical. Relax your shoulders, neck and spine.

Hold the charge in legs, arms, feet, hands, abdomen and chest with smooth rhythmic *Ujjayi* breathing, core of your body soft, till ready to return to *Trikonasana* on an **inhalation**, then turn and step back to *Tadasana* on an **exhalation**. **19** **25**

No. 24 Ardhaparsvattonasana

Spying Pose

This pose gives an intense stretch to both legs, while stimulating the feet. At the same time it lengthens the spine, releases the neck and clarifies the *bandhas*. It develops awareness of the relationship between the action of the legs and the quality and position of the pelvis. It is a preparation for *Parsvottanasana*.

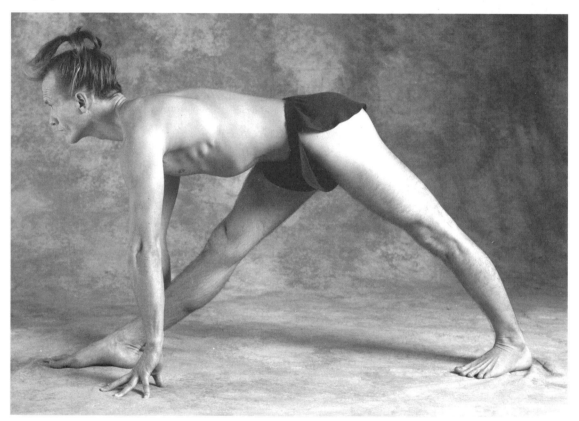

SUMMARY

With the feet wide apart, turn the front foot out 90 degrees, the back foot 75 degrees, and bring the back hip in line with the front, so the whole trunk is facing directly forwards. With straight legs, pivot the pelvis to bring the hands to the floor outside the front foot and extend the spine forwards looking ahead. Keep the arches of the feet lifting with the four corners pressing down equally, legs strong, pelvis even, *bandhas* engaged, core of the body soft with smooth rhythmic *Ujjayi* breathing.

28

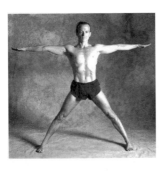

1 Start in *Tadasana*. As you **inhale**, turn to the right and step your feet wide apart, with your arms parallel to the floor. You are now in *Trikonasana*.

2 **Exhaling**, turn your right foot out 90 degrees and your left foot in 75 degrees, turning your whole leg with it. Line up the heel of your right foot with the ankle of your left foot.

3 **Inhaling**, turn your trunk with your legs to bring your left hip forward in line with the right, keeping your arms outstretched parallel to the floor.

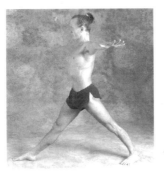

4 **Exhaling**, engage the legs fully, hitting the outer edge of your right knee back, the inner edge of your left knee back, while taking your left shin back into the calf and your right calf forward into the shin with the weight even between and across the surfaces of your feet.

5 **Inhaling**, broaden your ribcrest and suck your solar plexus in and up so your chest becomes active, broad and full, your abdomen passive, long and empty (*Uddiyanabandha*), and flatten your pubic abdomen, sucking your perineum and sacrum in with your anus soft (*Mulabandha*), keeping a strong charge in arms and legs.

133

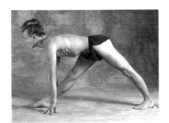

6 **Exhaling**, pivot your pelvis and keep your spine and trunk long as you take your fingertips to the floor on either side of your right foot.

7 **Inhaling**, extend your trunk and spine out of your pelvis, opening your chest as you look straight ahead.

Hold keeping the feet alive, legs strong, pelvis even, *bandhas* engaged, core of your body soft with smooth rhythmic *Ujjayi* breathing. Release by raising back up to *Trikonasana* on an **inhalation**.

Repeat to the left steps **2 to 7**, then turn and step back to *Tadasana* while **exhaling**. **28**

No. 25 Parsvottanasana

The Bowing Warrior Pose

This pose gives an intense stretch to both legs, while stimulating the feet. At the same time it challenges the *bandhas*. It develops awareness of the relationship between the action of the legs and the quality and position of the pelvis. It is both preparation and counter-pose to *Virabhadrasana*.

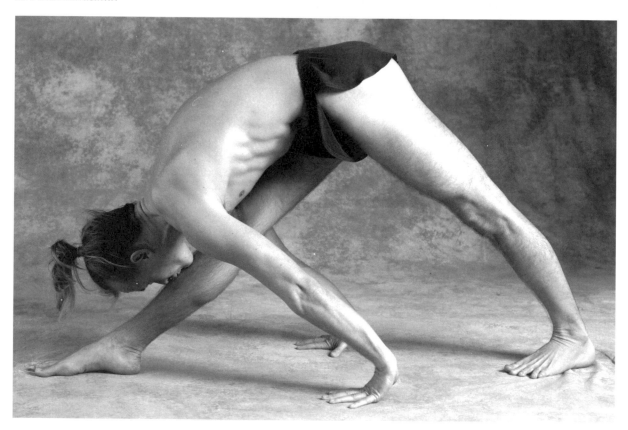

SUMMARY

With the feet wide apart turn the front foot out 90 degrees, the back foot 75 degrees, and bring the back hip in line with the front, so the whole trunk is facing directly forwards. With straight legs pivot the pelvis to bring the hands to the floor underneath the pelvis and extend the spine along the front leg, chin on the shin. Keep the arches of the feet lifting with the four corners pressing down equally, legs strong, pelvis even, *bandhas* engaged, core of the body soft with smooth rhythmic *Ujjayi* breathing.

26

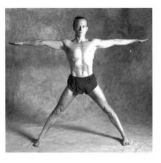

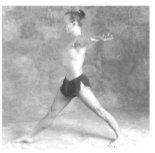

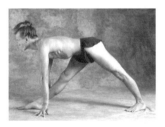

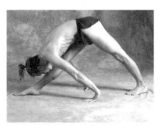

1 Start in *Tadasana*. As you **inhale**, turn to the right and step your feet wide apart, with your arms parallel to the floor. You are now in *Trikonasana*.

2 **Exhaling**, turn your right foot out 90 degrees and your left foot in 75 degrees, turning the whole leg with it. Line up the heel of your right foot with the ankle of your left foot.

3 **Inhaling**, turn your trunk with your legs to bring your left hip forward in line with the right, keeping your arms outstretched parallel to the floor.

4 **Exhaling**, engage the legs fully, hitting the outer edge of your right knee back, the inner edge of your left knee back, while taking your left shin back into the calf and your right calf forward into the shin with the weight even between and across the surfaces of your feet.

5 **Inhaling**, broaden your ribcrest and suck your solar plexus in and up so your chest becomes active, broad and full, your abdomen passive, long and empty (*Uddiyanabandha*), and flatten your pubic abdomen, sucking your perineum and sacrum in with your anus soft (*Mulabandha*), keeping a strong charge in arms and legs.

6 **Exhaling**, pivot your pelvis and keep your spine and trunk long as you take your fingertips to the floor on either side of your right foot.

7 **Inhaling**, extend your trunk and spine out of your pelvis, opening your chest.

8 **Exhaling**, keep your legs strong and your spine long as you extend your trunk along your right leg. Take your hands back and palms flat to the floor, and your chin to your shin.

Hold keeping the feet alive, legs strong, pelvis even, *bandhas* engaged, core of your body soft with smooth rhythmic *Ujjayi* breathing. Release by raising back up to *Trikonasana* on an **inhalation**.

Repeat to the left steps **2 to 8**, then turn and step back to *Tadasana* while **exhaling**. **26**

135

No. 26 Virabhadrasana

The Warrior Pose

This is an intense pose. It releases the pelvis and challenges the back leg and foot. Those with heart conditions should hold at Step **6** without raising the arms. It works on the spine like a backbend, and care must be taken to protect the lumbar vertebrae. This is done with the *bandhas* and keeping the back leg absolutely straight.

136

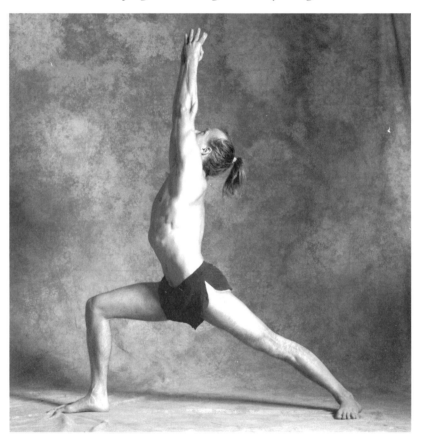

SUMMARY

With feet wide apart turn the legs and trunk to one side and raise the arms up gazing along the fingers. Bend the front leg 90 degrees, keeping the hips in line and the back leg strong. Keep the arches of the feet lifting with the four corners pressing down equally, *bandhas* engaged with abdomen long hollow and empty, chest broad and full, core of the body soft, with smooth rhythmic *Ujjayi* breathing. **27**

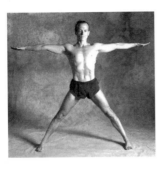

1 Start in *Tadasana*. As you **inhale**, turn to the right and step your feet wide apart, with your arms parallel to the floor. You are now in *Trikonasana*.

2 **Exhaling**, turn your right foot out 90 degrees and your left foot in 75 degrees, turning your whole leg with it. Line up the heel of your right foot with the ankle of your left foot.

3 **Inhaling**, turn your trunk with your legs to bring your left hip forward in line with the right, bringing your hands to your hips.

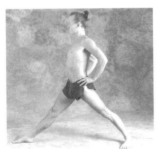

4 **Exhaling**, make your left leg strong, hitting the inner edge of your knee backwards and pressing your shinbone to your calf to keep the back of your knee open.

5 **Inhaling**, broaden your ribcrest and suck your solar plexus in and up so your chest becomes active, broad and full, your abdomen passive, long and empty (*Uddiyanabandha*), and flatten your pubic abdomen, sucking your perineum and sacrum in with your anus soft (*Mulabandha*), and extend your arms alongside your ears, keeping them straight, palms touching if they can.

137

6 **Exhaling**, bend your right leg to a right angle, thigh parallel to the floor, shin perpendicular, while keeping your left leg straight and strong.

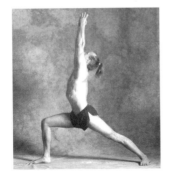

7 **Inhaling**, lift your right hip away from your thigh and suck your solar plexus in and up so your chest becomes active, broad and full, your abdomen passive, long and empty as you lengthen your spine and stretch your arms upwards, looking along your fingers.

Hold with your left leg strong and turning to keep the hip forwards, the weight even on your feet, *bandhas* engaged, core of your body soft, with smooth rhythmic *Ujjayi* breathing. Release to *Trikonasana* on an **inhalation**.

Repeat to the left steps **2 to 7**, then turn and step back to *Tadasana* while **exhaling**. **27**

No. 27 Parsvavirabhadrasana

Side Warrior Pose

This pose clarifies the importance of the pelvis and the spirallic nature of the line of force supporting *Asana*. This can be felt in the arms, legs and the hip sockets. It teaches the use of the back leg in resisting and supporting the action of the bent front leg.

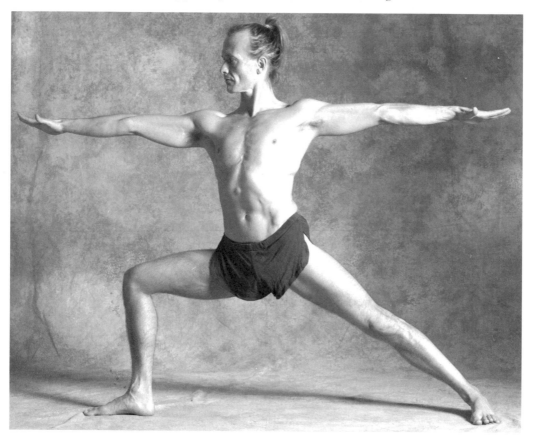

SUMMARY

Feet wide apart, extend the arms straight out of the armpits parallel to the floor and turn the front foot out 90 degrees, the back foot in 15/25 degrees. Bend the front leg to a right angle, resisting with the back leg. Keep the arches of the feet lifting with the four corners pressing down equally. Look along the front arm. Hold the charge in legs, arms, feet, hands, abdomen and chest with smooth rhythmic *Ujjayi* breathing, core of the body soft.

29

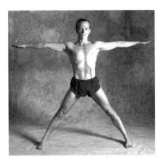

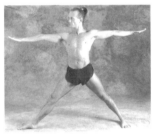

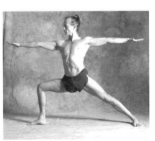

1 Start in *Tadasana*. As you **inhale**, turn to the right and step the feet wide apart, with your arms parallel to the floor. You are now in *Trikonasana*.

2 **Exhaling**, turn your right foot out 90 degrees and your left foot 15/25 degrees in without dropping the knee in. Line up the heel of your right foot with the ankle of your left foot.

3 **Inhaling**, broaden your ribcrest and suck your solar plexus in and up so your chest becomes active, broad and full, your abdomen passive, long and empty (*Uddiyanabandha*), and flatten your pubic abdomen, sucking your perineum and sacrum in with your anus soft (*Mulabandha*), keeping a strong charge in arms and legs.

4 **Exhaling**, sucking the thigh muscles in, hit the outer edge of your left knee backwards and roll your left hip backwards, while keeping the right buttock tucked in.

5 **Inhaling**, lengthen your spine and open your chest.

6 **Exhaling**, resist with the left leg by hitting the inner knee out, the outer knee back, and bend your right leg until you have a right angle, knee directly above the ankle, shin bone perpendicular, thigh bone parallel to the floor. Keep the arms charged and extending parallel to the floor, looking along your right hand.

Hold the charge in legs, arms, feet, hands, abdomen and chest with smooth rhythmic *Ujjayi* breathing, core of your body soft, till ready to return to *Trikonasana* on an **inhalation**.

Repeat steps **2 to 6**, then turn and step back to *Tadasana* on an **exhalation**. **29**

139

No. 28 Ekapadasana

Crane Pose

This pose develops balance and stability, and is a preparation for other more challenging leg-balancing poses. It teaches the importance of the ankles for balance.

SUMMARY

Standing on one straight strong leg, keep the spine long and raise the other knee higher than and in line with its hip. Keep the arch of the standing foot lifting with the four corners pressing down equally. Keep the *bandhas* engaged, abdomen long hollow and empty, chest broad and full, core of the body soft, with smooth rhythmic *Ujjayi* breathing. **32**

140

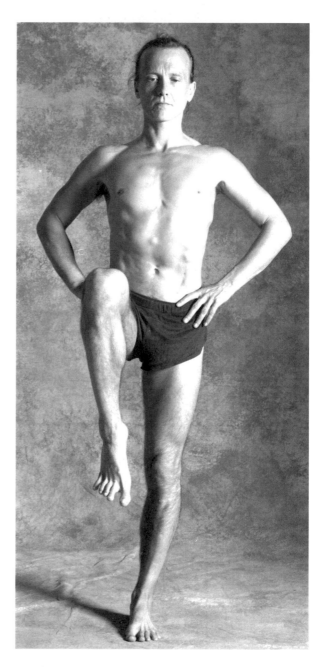

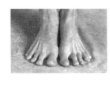

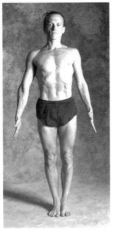

1 Stand upright with your feet together, touching at the inner heel and ball of the big toe, if possible. If not, keep the feet parallel to each other as close together as possible.

2 Spread your body weight evenly across both feet, so they bear the same weight. The heels and balls of your feet and the inner and outer edges of your feet should bear the same weight. Maintain a strong, clear contact between your inner ankles, so they do not roll apart or forwards. Feel the four corners of each foot – balls of the big and little toes and the inner and outer heels – pressing down with arches lifting.

3 **Exhaling**, suck the thigh muscles into the bones so that the backs of your knees open evenly and your legs and kneecaps are centred. Your kneecaps will automatically engage.

4 **Inhaling**, lift your armpits away from your hipbones, broaden your ribcrest, and suck your solar plexus in and up so your chest becomes active, broad and full, your abdomen passive, long and empty (*Uddiyanabandha*), and flatten your pubic abdomen, sucking your perineum and sacrum in with your anus soft (*Mulabandha*).

141

5 **Exhaling**, shift your body weight all on to the left foot while still keeping the right foot in position on the floor.

6 **Inhaling**, raise your right knee up as high as you comfortably can, keeping the knee and foot in line with your hip.

Hold with the left leg strong, spine long, *bandhas* engaged, core of your body soft, with smooth rhythmic *Ujjayi* breathing, until ready to release back to *Tadasana* on an **exhalation**.

Repeat steps **2 to 6** standing on the right leg, then return to *Tadasana*. **32**

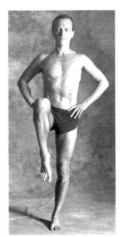

No. 29 Ekapadangustasana

Balancing Pose

This pose utilizes the dynamic of a triangle to straighten the spine and the raised leg. It develops balance and stability while strengthening legs and feet, balancing the pelvis and lengthening the spine and arms. It teaches the importance of the ankles for balance, and the importance of straightening the legs to support the spine.

142

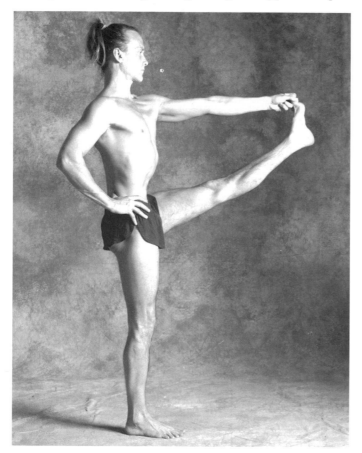

SUMMARY
Standing on one straight strong leg, keep the arch of the foot lifting with the four corners pressing down equally. Keep the spine long and raise and straighten the other leg in front of you, holding the big toe. Keep the *bandhas* engaged, abdomen long hollow and empty, chest broad and full, core of the body soft, with smooth rhythmic *Ujjayi* breathing.

30

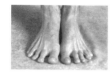

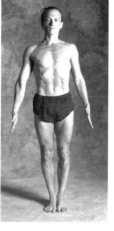

1 Stand upright with your feet together, touching at the inner heel and ball of the big toe, if possible. If not, keep the feet parallel to each other as close together as possible.

2 Spread your body weight evenly across both feet, so they bear the same weight. The heels and balls of the feet and the inner and outer edges of the feet should bear the same weight. Maintain a strong, clear contact between the inner ankles, so they do not roll apart or forwards. Feel the four corners of each foot – balls of the big and little toes and the inner and outer heels – pressing down with arches lifting.

3 **Exhaling**, suck the thigh muscles into the bones so that the backs of the knees open evenly and the legs and kneecaps are centred. Your kneecaps will automatically engage.

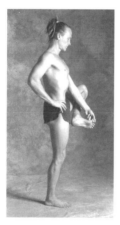

4 **Inhaling**, lift your armpits away from your hipbones, broaden your ribcrest, and suck your solar plexus in and up so your chest becomes active, broad and full, your abdomen passive, long and empty (*Uddiyanabandha*), and flatten your pubic abdomen, sucking your perineum and sacrum in with your anus soft (*Mulabandha*),

5 **Exhaling**, shift your body weight all on to the left foot while still keeping the right foot in position on the floor.

6 **Inhaling**, raise your right knee and catch the big toe with the thumb and two fingers of your right hand.

143

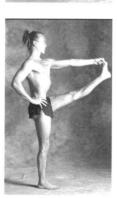

7 **Exhaling**, straighten your right leg forwards while keeping the left leg straight and strong – you may have to slide the hands down the shin to keep the leg straight.

Hold with the left leg strong, spine long, *bandhas* engaged, core of the body soft, with smooth rhythmic *Ujjayi* breathing, until ready to release back to *Tadasana* on an **exhalation** and repeat steps **2 to 7** standing on your right leg, finishing in *Tadasana*.

30

No. 30 Parsvaikapadangustasana

Side Balancing Pose

This pose utilizes the dynamic of a triangle to straighten the spine and the raised leg. It develops balance and stability while strengthening legs and feet, balancing the pelvis, opening the hip joints and lengthening the spine. It teaches the importance of the ankles for balance, and the importance of straightening the legs to support the spine.

144

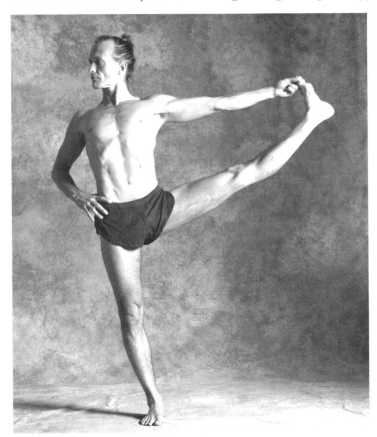

SUMMARY

Standing on one straight strong leg, keep the arch of the foot lifting with the four corners pressing down equally. Keep the spine long and raise and straighten the other leg to its side, holding the big toe, turning the head the other way. Keep the *bandhas* engaged, abdomen long hollow and empty, chest broad and full, core of the body soft, with smooth rhythmic *Ujjayi* breathing. **31**

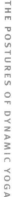

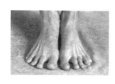

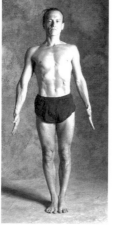

1   Stand upright with your feet together, touching at the inner heel and ball of the big toe, if possible. If not, keep the feet parallel to each other as close together as possible.

2   Spread your body weight evenly across both feet, so they bear the same weight. The heels and balls of the feet and the inner and outer edges of the feet should bear the same weight. Maintain a strong, clear contact between your inner ankles, so they do not roll apart or forwards. Feel the four corners of each foot – balls of the big and little toes and the inner and outer heels – pressing down with arches lifting.

3   **Exhaling**, suck your thigh muscles into your bones so that the backs of your knees open evenly and your legs and kneecaps are centred. Your kneecaps will automatically engage.

4   **Inhaling**, lift your armpits away from your hipbones, broaden your ribcrest, and suck your solar plexus in and up so your chest becomes active, broad and full, your abdomen passive, long and empty (*Uddiyanabandha*), and flatten your pubic abdomen, sucking your perineum and sacrum in with your anus soft (*Mulabandha*).

145

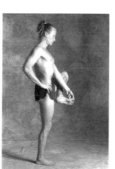

5   **Exhaling**, shift your body weight all on to the left foot while still keeping the right foot in position on the floor.

6   **Inhaling**, raise your right knee and catch the big toe with the thumb and two fingers of your right hand.

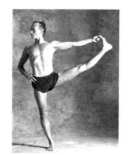

7   **Exhaling**, straighten your right leg to its side while keeping your left leg straight and strong – you may have to slide your hands down the shin to keep the leg straight. Turn your head to the left.

Hold with the left leg strong, spine long, *bandhas* engaged, core of your body soft, with smooth rhythmic *Ujjayi* breathing, until ready to release back to *Tadasana* on an **exhalation**, and repeat steps **2 to 7** standing on the right leg, then return to *Tadasana*.

31

No. 31 Vriksasana

Tree Pose

This pose develops stability and balance, while opening the hip joint and stabilizing the sacrum. It develops quietness of mind.

146

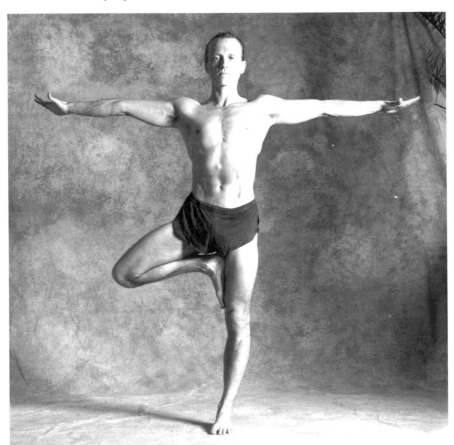

SUMMARY

Standing on one straight strong leg, keep the arch of the foot lifting with the four corners pressing down equally. Keep the spine long and place the other foot high in the centre of the straight leg thigh, knee kept back, and extend the arms parallel to the floor. Keep the *bandhas* engaged, abdomen long hollow and empty, chest broad and full, core of the body soft, with smooth rhythmic *Ujjayi* breathing.

32

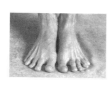

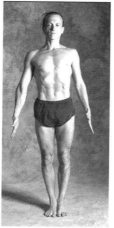

1 Stand upright with your feet together, touching at the inner heel and ball of the big toe, if possible. If not, keep the feet parallel to each other as close together as possible.

2 Spread your body weight evenly across both feet, so they bear the same weight. The heels and balls of the feet and the inner and outer edges of the feet should bear the same weight. Maintain a strong, clear contact between your inner ankles, so they do not roll apart or forwards. Feel the four corners of each foot – balls of the big and little toes and the inner and outer heels – pressing down with arches lifting.

3 **Exhaling**, suck your thigh muscles into your bones so that your backs of your knees open evenly and your legs and kneecaps are centred. Your kneecaps will automatically engage.

4 **Inhaling**, lift your armpits away from your hipbones, broaden your ribcrest, and suck your solar plexus in and up so your chest becomes active, broad and full, your abdomen passive, long and empty (*Uddiyanabandha*), and flatten your pubic abdomen, sucking your perineum and sacrum in with your anus soft (*Mulabandha*).

5 **Exhaling**, shift your body weight all on to the left foot while still keeping the left foot in position on the floor.

6 **Inhaling**, raise your right knee and catch the ankle.

7 **Exhaling**, bend your right leg and place the foot on high to the centre of the inner left thigh, while keeping your left leg straight and strong.

8 **Inhaling**, extend your arms parallel to the floor.

9 **Exhaling**, press your right foot hard into the resisting left leg and, without turning your pelvis or spine, draw your right knee back and take your sacrum in.

Hold with the left leg strong, spine long, *bandhas* engaged, core of your body soft, with smooth rhythmic *Ujjayi* breathing, until ready to release back to *Tadasana* on an **exhalation**, and repeat steps **2 to 9** standing on the right leg, and return back to *Tadasana*.

32

147

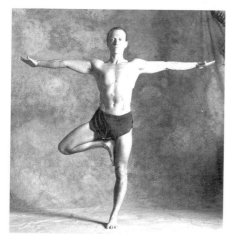

No. 32 Dandasana

The Staff

This pose is the basic sitting pose. Simple but challenging. When tired it can be held for a few breaths instead of an active *vinyasa* in between poses. It awakens the whole body, develops the legs, releases the pelvis and the spine. Preparation for forward extensions. Preparation of the spine for meditation. It teaches the meaning of dynamic stillness.

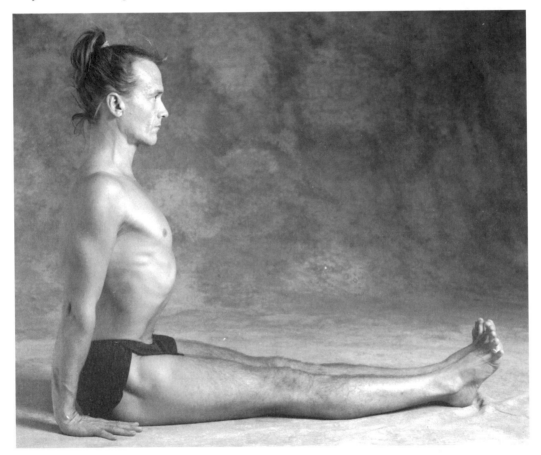

SUMMARY

Sit with legs together outstretched, straight and strong. Activate the *bandhas* to elevate the spine out of the pelvis while pressing the palms down outside the buttocks, abdomen long hollow and empty, chest broad and full. Keep feet, hands, legs and arms alive with smooth, rhythmic *Ujjayi* breathing, core of the body soft. ✦ 33 38

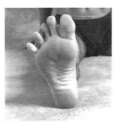

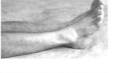

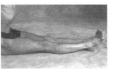

1 Sit on the floor with legs outstretched, but relaxed in front of you. Make sure your pelvis and trunk are not twisted, bringing the inner heels in line against each other.

2 Roll the inner ankles together and join the inner edges of your feet so that the balls of the big toes touch.

3 Lengthen from the inner ankle to the inner heel and broaden the ball of your foot so that your calf muscles suck into the shinbone.

4 Lengthen your front ankle without shortening the Achilles tendon, and extend your toes towards the ceiling. Keep the ball of your foot the furthest part of you from the spine.

5 **Exhaling**, bring the backs of your knees to the floor by sucking your thigh muscles in to the bone. At the same time, bring your hipbones slightly forwards of the buttock bones.

6 **Inhaling**, broaden your ribcrest, sucking your solar plexus in and up so your chest becomes active, broad and full, your abdomen passive, long and empty (*Uddiyanabandha*) while at the same time flattening your pubic abdomen, sucking your perineum and sacrum in with anus soft (*Mulabandha*). Keep the core of your body soft as your spine lengthens out of your pelvis.

149

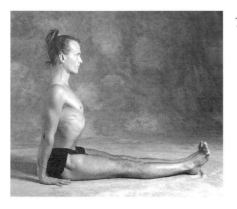

7 **Exhaling**, press your palms into the floor by your buttocks, arms straight. Relax your shoulders and tuck your shoulder blades in. Look straight ahead.

Hold till ready to release on an **inhalation**, and follow the breath through one of the *vinyasa* sequences to the next posture indicated below, for the Series you are practising. ✸ 33 38

No. 33 Urdhvaikapadasana

Raised Leg Pose

Be careful of the bent-leg knee. It challenges *Uddiyanabandha*. This pose awakens the feet and legs, strengthening the spine and back muscles, while mobilizing the hip sockets. It teaches the relationship between the action of the limbs and the quality of the spine. This pose can be done alone or as part of a single flow of *Urdhvaikapadasana* (**33**), *Parsvaikapadasana* (**34**), *Parivrttaikapadasana* (**35**), *Ekapadanavasana* (**36**), and *Sukhapascimottanasana* (**37**), all done with the left leg, then through a *vinyasa* to repeat with the right leg. Wait until you are comfortable with each pose individually before practising this way.

150

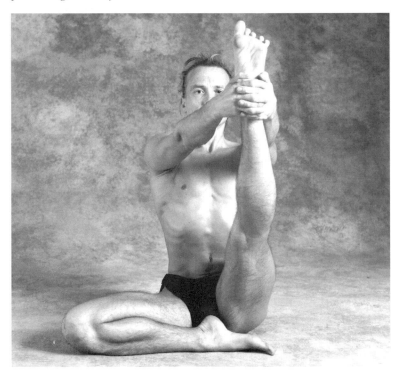

SUMMARY

Sitting on both buttocks, bend one leg in to the opposite buttock then take the heel of the other leg with both hands and straighten the leg upwards directly in front of you. Keep the spine long, the straight leg and its foot charged, the core of the body soft, while maintaining the *bandhas* with the abdomen long, hollow and empty, the chest broad and full with smooth rhythmic *Ujjayi* breathing. ✦ 34 34

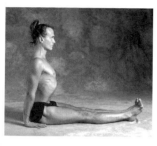

1   Sit on the floor with legs outstretched, straight and strong, feet together and alive, with your spine lifting straight out of your pelvis (*Dandasana*).

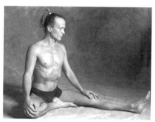

2   **Exhaling**, bend your right leg so that your right foot touches the top, inner left thigh.

3   **Inhaling**, bend your left leg and take hold of the heel with both hands, keeping it in line with the buttock.

4   **Exhaling**, straighten your left leg upwards directly in front of you.

5   **Inhaling**, lift and broaden your ribcrest, sucking your solar plexus in and up so your chest becomes active, broad and full, your abdomen passive, long and empty (*Uddiyanabandha*) and flatten your pubic abdomen, with your anus soft as you suck your perineum and sacrum in (*Mulabandha*).

151

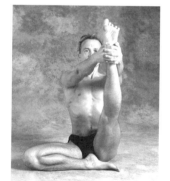

6   **Exhaling**, use your hands to lift your trunk higher and longer against the stability of the straight left leg, as you look straight ahead.

Hold, with your left leg strong, foot alive, core of your body soft, maintaining the *bandhas* with smooth, rhythmic *Ujjayi* breathing, till ready to **exhale** and take the leg to the side right-hand to its hip to *Parsvaikapadasana* (**34**) steps **4 to 6**.

IF BEING DONE SEPARATELY, **inhaling** to *Dandasana* and following the breath through one of the short *vinyasa* sequences, and then repeat steps **2 to 6** on the other side. When you have done both sides follow the breath through any of the *vinyasa* sequences to *Parsvaikapadasana* (**34**). 34 34

No. 34 Parsvaikapadasana

Side Raised Leg Pose

Be careful of the bent-leg knee. This pose awakens the feet and legs, while mobilizing the hip sockets and refining the *bandhas*. This pose can be done alone or as part of a single flow of *Urdhvaikapadasana* (**33**), *Parsvaikapadasana* (**34**), *Parivrttaikapadasana* (**35**), *Ekapadanavasana* (**36**), and *Sukhapascimottanasana* (**37**), all done with the left leg, then through a *vinyasa* to repeat with the right leg. Wait until you are comfortable with each pose individually before practising this way.

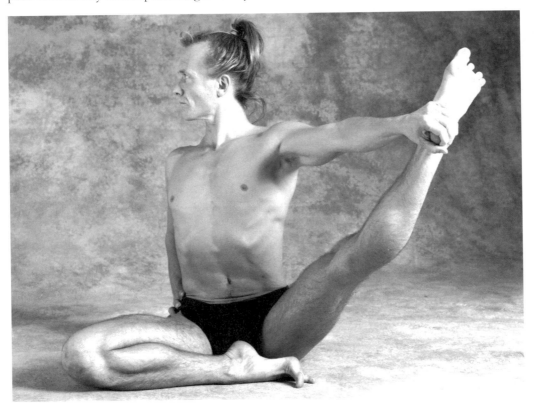

SUMMARY

Sitting on both buttocks, bend one leg into the opposite buttock then take the inner heel of the other leg with its hand and straighten the leg wide to the side of you, while looking over the other shoulder. Keep the spine long, the straight leg and its foot charged, the core of the body soft, while maintaining the *bandhas* with the abdomen long, hollow and empty, the chest broad and full with smooth, rhythmic *Ujjayi* breathing.

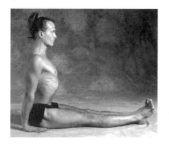

1 Sit on the floor with legs outstretched, straight and strong, feet together and alive, with your spine lifting straight out of your pelvis (*Dandasana*).

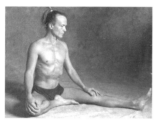

2 **Exhaling**, bend your right leg so that your right foot touches the top, inner left thigh.

3 **Inhaling**, bend your left leg and take hold of the inner heel with your left hand, and put your right hand on your right hip, or on the floor beside your right buttock.

4 **Exhaling**, straighten your left leg upwards, wide to the left of you.

153

5 **Inhaling**, lift and broaden your ribcrest, sucking your solar plexus in and up so your chest becomes active, broad and full, your abdomen passive, long and empty (*Uddiyanabandha*) and flatten your pubic abdomen, with your anus soft as you suck your perineum and sacrum in (*Mulabandha*).

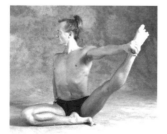

6 **Exhaling**, use your left hand to lift the trunk higher and longer against the stability of the straight left leg, as you look to the right.

Hold, with the left leg strong, foot alive, core of the body soft, maintaining the *bandhas* with smooth, rhythmic *Ujjayi* breathing, till ready to **exhale** and cross the leg over the body into the other hand, free hand onto its hip, into *Parivrttaika-padasana* (**35**) steps **4 to 6**.

IF BEING DONE SEPARATELY, **inhaling** to *Dandasana* and following the breath through one of the short *vinyasa* sequences, and then repeat steps **2 to 6** on the other side. When you have done both sides, follow the breath through any of the *vinyasa* sequences to *Parivrttaikapadasana* (**35**). ✴ **35**

No. 35 Parivrttaikapadasana

Twisting Raised Leg Pose

Be careful of the bent-leg knee. This pose awakens the feet and legs, softens the spine and back muscles, while mobilizing the hip sockets, sacrum and sacroiliac joints. This pose can be done alone or as part of a single flow of *Urdhvaikapadasana* (**33**), *Parsvaikapadasana* (**34**), *Parivrttaikapadasana* (**35**), *Ekapadanavasana* (**36**), and *Sukhapascimottanasana* (**37**), all done with the left leg, then through a *vinyasa* to repeat with the right leg. Wait until you are comfortable with each pose individually before practising this way.

154

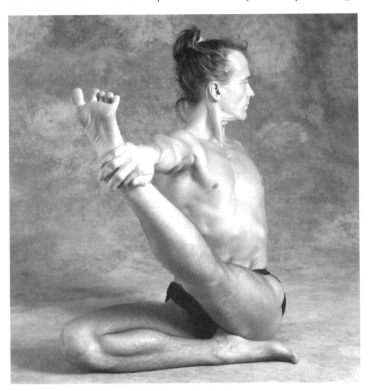

SUMMARY

Sitting on both buttocks, bend one leg into the opposite buttock, then take the outer heel of the other leg with the opposite hand and straighten and lift the leg across the line of your body while turning your head the other way. Keep the spine long, the straight leg and its foot charged, the core of the body soft, while maintaining the *bandhas* with the abdomen long, hollow and empty, the chest broad and full with smooth, rhythmic *Ujjayi* breathing. 37 36

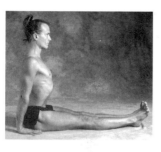

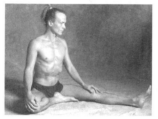

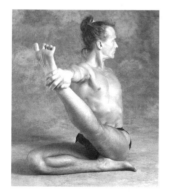

1 Sit on the floor with legs outstretched, straight and strong, feet together and alive, with your spine lifting straight out of your pelvis (*Dandasana*).

2 **Exhaling**, bend your right leg so that your right foot touches the top, inner left thigh.

3 **Inhaling**, bend your left leg and take hold of the outer heel with your right hand, and put your left hand on your left hip or on the floor by your buttock.

4 **Exhaling**, straighten your left leg upwards and draw it across the line of your body, while turning your head the other way, to the left and rolling your left shoulder back.

5 **Inhaling**, lift and broaden your ribcrest, sucking your solar plexus in and up so your chest becomes active, broad and full, your abdomen passive, long and empty (*Uddiyanabandha*) and flatten your pubic abdomen, with your anus soft as you suck your perineum and sacrum in (*Mulabandha*).

155

6 **Exhaling**, use your right hand to lift your trunk higher and longer against the stability of the straight left leg, as you look to the left.

Hold, with the left leg strong, foot alive, core of the body soft, maintaining the *bandhas* with smooth, rhythmic *Ujjayi* breathing, till ready to **exhale** and bring the leg to centre and, in the Foundation Series, hands to the hips into *Ekapadanavasana* (**36**) step **7** or, in the Pacifying Series, bring the left thigh down on to the arch of the right foot and follow *Sukhapascimottanasana* (**37**) steps **3 to 8**.

IF BEING DONE SEPARATELY, **inhaling** to *Dandasana* and following the breath through one of the short *vinyasa* sequences, and then repeat steps **2 to 6** on the other side. When you have done both sides, follow the breath through any of the *vinyasa* sequences to the next posture indicated below, for the Series you are practising. ✴ 36

No. 36 Ekapadanavasana

Single Legged Boat

This pose strengthens the legs and back. Preparation for *Navasana*. It refines the use of *Uddiyanabandha*. It teaches to hold the leg straight and unsupported without tightening the abdomen, and the importance of the feet in engaging the legs. This pose can be done alone or as part of a single flow of *Urdhvaikapadasana* (**33**), *Parsvaikapadasana* (**34**), *Parivrttaikapadasana* (**35**), *Ekapadanavasana* (**36**), and *Sukhapascimottanasana* (**37**), all done with the left leg, then through a *vinyasa* to repeat with the right leg. Wait until you are comfortable with each pose individually before practising this way.

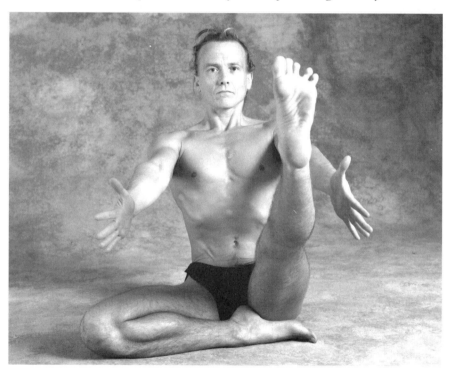

156

SUMMARY

Sitting on both buttocks, bend one leg into the opposite buttock, then take the heel of the other leg with both hands and straighten the leg upwards directly in front of you, then let go of the heel and extend the arms parallel to the floor on each side of the leg. Keep the spine long, the straight leg and its foot charged, the core of the body soft, while maintaining the *bandhas* with the abdomen long, hollow and empty, the chest broad and full with smooth, rhythmic *Ujjayi* breathing.

37

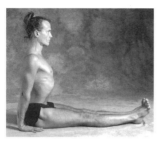

1 Sit on the floor with legs outstretched, straight and strong, feet together and alive, with your spine lifting straight out of your pelvis (*Dandasana*).

2 **Exhaling**, bend your right leg so that your right foot touches the top, inner left thigh.

3 **Inhaling**, bend your left leg and take hold of the heel with both hands, keeping it in line with your buttock.

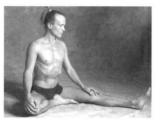

4 **Exhaling**, straighten your left leg upwards directly in front of you.

5 **Inhaling**, lift and broaden your ribcrest, sucking your solar plexus in and up so your chest becomes active, broad and full, your abdomen passive, long and empty (*Uddiyanabandha*) and flatten your pubic abdomen, with your anus soft as you suck your perineum and sacrum in (*Mulabandha*).

157

6 **Exhaling**, use your hands to lift the trunk higher and longer against the stability of the straight left leg, as you look straight ahead.

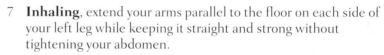

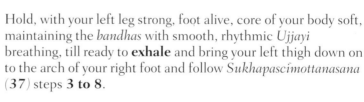

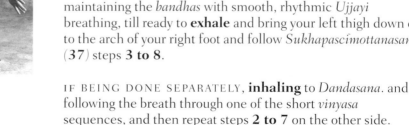

7 **Inhaling**, extend your arms parallel to the floor on each side of your left leg while keeping it straight and strong without tightening your abdomen.

Hold, with your left leg strong, foot alive, core of your body soft, maintaining the *bandhas* with smooth, rhythmic *Ujjayi* breathing, till ready to **exhale** and bring your left thigh down on to the arch of your right foot and follow *Sukhapascimottanasana* (*37*) steps **3 to 8**.

IF BEING DONE SEPARATELY, **inhaling** to *Dandasana*. and following the breath through one of the short *vinyasa* sequences, and then repeat steps **2 to 7** on the other side. When you have done both sides, follow the breath through any of the *vinyasa* sequences to *Sukhapascimottanasana* (*37*).

37

No. 37 Sukhapascimottanasana

Easy Forward Extension

This pose resembles the action of *Padmasana* in the bent leg, without utilizing the twist in the knee required of lifting into *Padmasana*, which is too much for many a sedentary knee to bear. Nevertheless care must be taken that there is no pain in the bent-leg knee. If there is, straighten the leg at right angles to the other one, and continue. It promotes internalization and challenges *Uddiyanabandha*. It releases tension from the spine and back, and opens the joints of the legs. It teaches the importance of the feet in engaging the legs. This pose can be done alone or as part of a single flow of *Urdhvaikapadasana* (**33**), *Parsvaikapadasana* (**34**), *Parivrttaikapadasana* (**35**), *Ekapadanavasana* (**36**), and *Sukhapascimottanasana* (**37**), all done with the left leg, then through a *vinyasa* to repeat with the right leg. Wait until you are comfortable with each pose individually before practising this way.

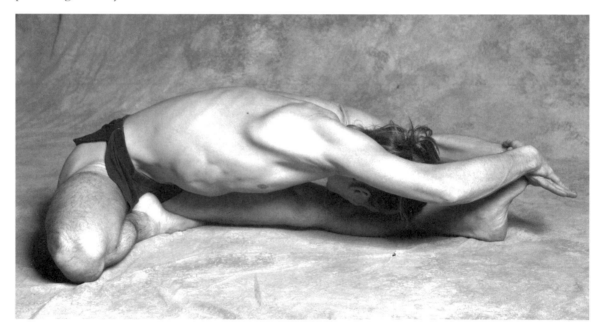

SUMMARY

With one leg straight and the other bent with the foot under the other thigh heel against the pubis, extend the spine forwards and down along the straight leg. Relaxing the spine and neck, charge the straight leg and foot. Core of the body soft, maintain the *bandhas* with the abdomen long, hollow and empty, the chest broad and full, with smooth, rhythmic *Ujjayi* breathing. ⭐47 43

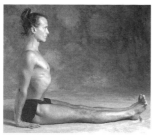

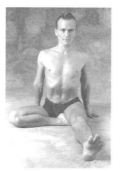

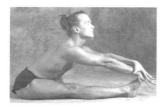

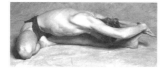

1 Sit on the floor with legs outstretched, straight and strong, feet together and alive, with your spine lifting straight out of your pelvis (*Dandasana*).

2 Bending your right leg, slightly raise your left thigh and slip your right foot under so that your left thigh rests on the arch of your right foot, while your right heel touches the centre of your pubic bone. Relax your right leg completely.

3 **Exhaling**, extend your left leg, broaden the ball of the foot, lengthen the inner heel and front ankle and suck the thigh muscles in so the back of the knee goes down as your leg straightens.

4 **Inhaling**, lift and broaden your ribcrest, sucking your solar plexus in and up so your chest becomes active, broad and full, your abdomen passive, long and empty (*Uddiyanabandha*) and flatten your pubic abdomen, with your anus soft as you suck your perineum and sacrum in (*Mulabandha*).

5 **Exhaling**, pivot your pelvis and reach forward with both hands and catch your left shin, ankle or foot, keeping your left leg straight, the foot alive.

6 **Inhaling**, clarify the *bandhas* as you lift your chin, lengthen the front of your spine and open your chest, keeping your left leg straight.

7 **Exhaling**, bend your arms, drawing your elbows forward, and lengthen the front of your spine forwards as it comes down towards the leg and relax your neck. Keep your left leg straight.

8 **Inhaling**, clarify the *bandhas* as you draw the crown of your head forward, lengthen the front of your spine and open your chest, keeping your left leg straight.

159

Hold, with the left leg strong, foot alive, core of the body soft, maintaining the *bandhas* with smooth, rhythmic *Ujjayi* breathing, till ready to release while keeping the charge of the *bandhas* and the leg **inhaling** to *Dandasana*. Then follow the breath through one of the short *vinyasa* sequences, and then repeat steps **2 to 8** on the other side. When you have done both sides, follow the breath through any of the *vinyasa* sequences to the next posture indicated, for the Series you are practising.

Done dynamically, by repeating steps **6 and 7**, this pose gently softens the back and hamstrings. ✴ 43

No. 38 Ekapadapascimottanasana

One Leg Forward Extension

This pose is the simplest forward bend. Nevertheless care must be taken that there is no pain in the bent-leg knee. If there is, straighten the leg at right angles to the other one, and continue. It promotes internalization and challenges *Uddiyanabandha*. It releases tension from the spine and back, and opens the joints of the legs. It teaches the importance of the feet in engaging the legs.

160

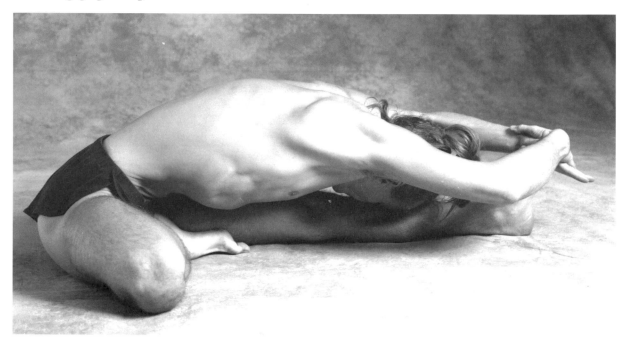

SUMMARY

With one leg straight and the other bent with the foot against the opposite leg, heel in the groin, extend the spine forwards and down along the straight leg. Relaxing the spine and neck, charge the straight leg and foot. Core of the body soft, maintain the *bandhas* with the abdomen long, hollow and empty, the chest broad and full with smooth, rhythmic *Ujjayi* breathing. **39**

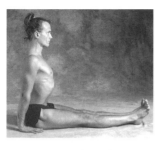

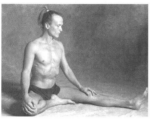

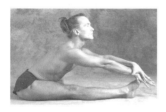

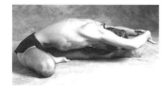

1 Sit on the floor with legs outstretched, straight and strong, feet together and alive, with your spine lifting straight out of your pelvis (*Dandasana*).

2 Bending your right leg, place your right foot against the top inner left thigh, heel into the groin. Relax your right leg completely.

3 **Exhaling**, extend your left leg, broadening the ball of your foot, lengthening the inner heel and front ankle and sucking the thigh muscles in so the back of your knee goes down as your leg straightens.

4 **Inhaling**, lift and broaden your ribcrest, sucking your solar plexus in and up so your chest becomes active, broad and full, your abdomen passive, long and empty (*Uddiyanabandha*) and flatten your pubic abdomen, with your anus soft as you suck your perineum and sacrum in (*Mulabandha*).

5 **Exhaling**, pivot your pelvis and reach forward with both hands and catch the left shin, ankle or foot, keeping your left leg straight, the foot alive.

6 **Inhaling**, clarify the *bandhas* as you lift your chin, lengthen your front of your spine and open your chest, keeping your left leg straight.

7 **Exhaling**, bend your arms, drawing the elbows forward, and lengthen the front of your spine forwards as it comes down towards the leg, neck relaxed. Keep your left leg straight.

8 **Inhaling**, clarify the *bandhas* as you draw the crown of your head forward, lengthen the front of your spine and open your chest, keeping your left leg straight.

Hold, with the left leg strong, foot alive, core of the body soft, maintaining the *bandhas* with smooth, rhythmic *Ujjayi* breathing, till ready to release while keeping the charge of the *bandhas* and the leg, **inhaling** to *Dandasana*. Then follow the breath through one of the short *vinyasa* sequences, and then repeat steps **2 to 8** on the other side. When you have done both sides, follow the breath through any of the *vinyasa* sequences to the *Padmapascimottanasana* (**39**).

Done dynamically, by repeating steps **6 and 7**, this pose gently softens the back and hamstrings.

39

No. 39 Padmapascimottanasana

Lotus Forward Extension

This pose releases the hip, knee and ankle joint while working deep into the hip socket, sacroiliac joint and the pelvic ligaments. It teaches the importance of straight legs to forward extensions. Preparation for *Padmasana*. Care must be taken that there is no pain in the bent-leg knee. If there is, straighten the leg at right angles to the other one, and continue. If half-lotus is not possible, but you have no pain in the knee, place the foot under the opposite thigh so that its leg makes the same shape and angle as it would in Lotus. (Please refer to Posture No. 37, *Sukhapadapascimottanasana*.)

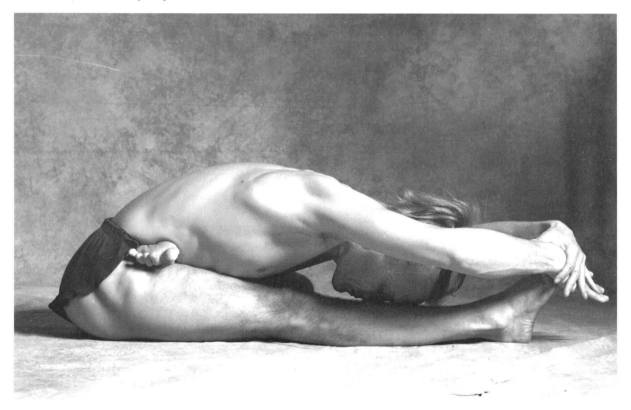

SUMMARY

With one leg straight and the other in half-lotus, extend the spine forwards and down along the straight leg. Relaxing the spine and neck, charge the straight leg and foot. Core of the body soft, maintain the *bandhas* with the abdomen long, hollow and empty, the chest broad and full with smooth, rhythmic *Ujjayi* breathing.

40

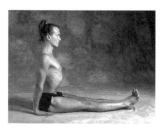

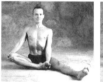 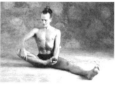

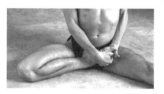

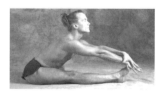

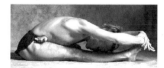

1 Sit on the floor with legs outstretched, straight and strong, feet together and alive, with your spine lifting straight out of your pelvis (*Dandasana*).

2 Relax your legs and take hold of your right leg by the knee and the heel, keeping it relaxed. Supporting the weight of the leg by the heel, use your right hand to pull the flesh of the calf and thigh up towards you so that the bones of the thigh and shin can come closer together. Use both hands to bring the shin bone as tight against the thigh bone as possible, making sure you do not twist the shin up towards your face.

3 Move the right thigh close to the left, and as the right foot draws near the left thigh, place it on top of the thigh with the heel near your navel.

4 **Exhaling**, extend your left leg, broaden the ball of the foot, lengthen the inner heel and front ankle and suck the thigh muscles in so the back of your knee goes down, leg straight.

5 **Inhaling**, lift and broaden your ribcrest, sucking your solar plexus in and up so your chest becomes active, broad and full, your abdomen passive, long and empty (*Uddiyanabandha*) and flatten your pubic abdomen, with your anus soft as you suck your perineum and sacrum in (*Mulabandha*).

6 **Exhaling**, pivot your pelvis and reach forward with both hands and catch the left shin, ankle or foot, keeping the left leg straight, the foot alive.

7 **Inhaling**, clarify the *bandhas* as you lift your chin, lengthen the front of the spine and open the chest, keep the left leg straight.

8 **Exhaling**, bend your arms, drawing the elbows forward, and lengthen the front of your spine forwards as it comes down towards the leg, neck relaxed. Keep your left leg straight.

9 **Inhaling**, clarify the *bandhas* as you draw the crown of your head forward, lengthen the front of your spine and open your chest, keeping your left leg straight.

Hold with the *bandhas*, leg and foot alive, core soft, breath smooth, till ready to release to *Dandasana*. Then follow the breath through a *vinyasa*, repeating steps **2 to 9** on the other side. Then breathe through a *vinyasa* to *Janusirsasana* (**40**).

Done dynamically, by repeating steps **7 and 8**, this pose gently softens the back and hamstrings.

163

40

No. 40 Janusirsasana

Intense Forward Extension Pose

This gives the greatest stretch to the trunk of the forward extensions, in doing so it flushes the kidneys. Care must be taken that there is no pain in the bent-leg knee. If there is, straighten the leg at right angles to the other one, and continue. It promotes internalization and challenges *Uddiyanabandha*. It teaches the need to distinguish clearly between the opposing actions of each part of the body especially in and around the back hip. As in all these forward extensions, when the legs are fully engaged and the pelvis mobilized, the head comes to the shin almost at the ankle, not the knee. It works deep into the hip sockets, the sacroiliac joints and the pelvic ligaments.

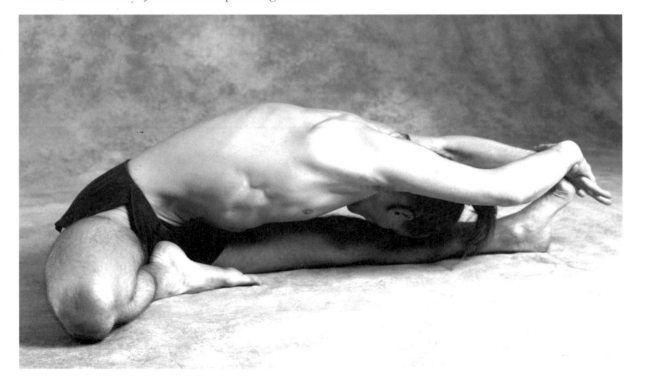

SUMMARY
With one leg straight and the other bent with the heel in its own groin so the knee is behind the line of the hips, extend the spine forwards and down along the straight leg. Relaxing the spine and neck charge the straight leg and foot. Core of the body soft, maintain the *bandhas* with the abdomen long, hollow and empty, the chest broad and full with smooth, rhythmic *Ujjayi* breathing.

41

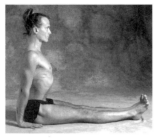

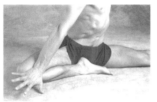

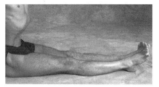

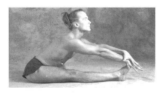

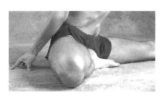

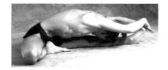

1 Sit on the floor with legs outstretched, straight and strong, feet together and alive, with your spine lifting straight out of your pelvis (*Dandasana*).

2 Bending your right knee, place the right heel in its own groin, so that your right knee is behind the line of the hips. Keep the ball of your right foot open, leg engaged.

3 **Exhaling**, extend your left leg, broaden the ball of the foot, lengthen the inner heel and front ankle and suck the thigh muscles in so the back of the knee goes down as the leg straightens.

4 **Inhaling**, lift and broaden your ribcrest, sucking your solar plexus in and up so your chest becomes active, broad and full, your abdomen passive, long and empty (*Uddiyanabandha*) and flatten your pubic abdomen, with your anus soft as you suck your perineum and sacrum in (*Mulabandha*).

5 **Exhaling**, pivot your pelvis and reach forward with both hands and catch the left shin, ankle or foot, keeping the left leg straight, the foot alive.

6 **Inhaling**, clarify the *bandhas* as you lift your chin, lengthen the front of the spine, open your chest, keep the left leg straight.

7 **Exhaling**, bend your arms, drawing the elbows forward, and lengthen the front of your spine forwards as it comes down towards the leg. Keep the left leg straight. Make sure you do not drag the right knee forward, but roll the top of the thigh forward as the shin bone tucks under and the knee centres. Create resistance in the knee so that it stays centred and the movement all comes in the trunk and pelvis. Relax the neck.

8 **Inhaling**, clarify the *bandhas* as you draw the crown of your head forward, lengthen the front of your spine and open your chest, keeping your left leg straight. Observe the position of the right knee, behind the line of the hips.

Hold with the *bandhas*, leg and foot alive, core soft, breath smooth, till ready to release to *Dandasana*. Then follow the breath through a *vinyasa*, repeating steps **2 to 8** on the other side. Then breathe through a *vinyasa* to *Marichyasana* (**41**).

Done dynamically, by repeating steps **6 and 7**, this pose gently softens the back and hamstrings. **41**

No. 41 Marichyasana

Marichya's Pose

This pose, and all others with one foot drawn in with the knee up, is named after the sage *Marichya*. It works deep into the hip socket, pelvic ligaments and lower back, while challenging the *bandhas*. It releases the neck and strengthens the wrists. The arms are used to support the back.

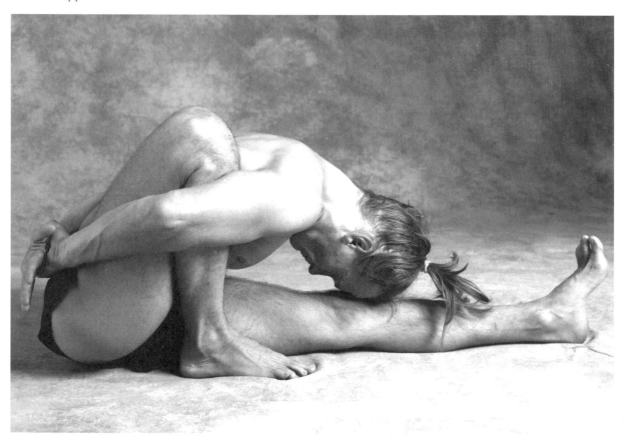

SUMMARY

Sitting with one leg straight, one bent with the foot in and knee up, wrap its own arm round the upright shin and catch the other hand behind the waist. Keeping the spine long, extend it along the straight leg and relax the spine, shoulders and neck keeping the feet and legs active. Maintain the *bandhas* with the abdomen long, hollow and empty, the chest broad and full, core of the body soft, with smooth, rhythmic *Ujjayi* breathing. **42**

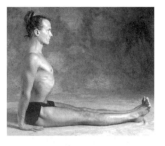

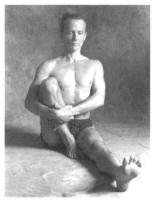

1 Sit on the floor with legs outstretched, straight and strong, feet together and alive, with your spine lifting straight out of your pelvis (*Dandasana*).

2 **Exhaling**, bend your right leg by drawing the foot into your pubis, keeping the knee straight up and catch hold of the right shin with both hands. Keep pressing your right foot firmly into the floor so the calf and thigh engage, right foot against left thigh.

3 **Inhaling**, lift and broaden your ribcrest, sucking your solar plexus in and up so your chest becomes active, broad and full, your abdomen passive, long and empty (*Uddiyanabandha*) and flatten your pubic abdomen, with your anus soft as you suck your perineum and sacrum in (*Mulabandha*).

4 **Exhaling**, release your right hand and extend your right arm forward to catch your right foot or ankle, while pulling low down on your right shin with your left hand.

5 **Inhaling**, lift and lengthen your spine.

6 **Exhaling**, lengthen your right arm and, keeping it straight and long, pull it back against your right shin so that your shin is in your armpit, not lower down your arm.

7 **Inhaling**, lift and lengthen your spine.

8 **Exhaling**, bend your right arm back around your shin to catch your left hand behind your waist.

9 **Inhaling**, lift and lengthen your spine.

10 **Exhaling**, extend your trunk forward along your left leg, using your right arm against your shin bone as a lever to propel your spine forwards as you come down towards the leg. Relax your neck.

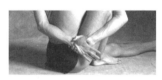

167

Hold with your left leg strong, right foot pressing the floor, neck, shoulders and spine relaxed, core of your body soft, *bandhas* engaged, with smooth, rhythmic *Ujjayi* breathing until ready to release back to *Dandasana* on an **inhalation**, maintaining the *bandhas*, and follow the breath through one of the short *vinyasa* sequences, and then repeat steps **2 to 10** on the other side. When you have done both sides, follow the breath through any of the *vinyasa* sequences to *Sukhamarichyasana* (**42**). **42**

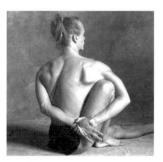

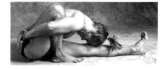

No. 42 Sukhamarichyasana

Easy Marichya's Pose

This pose can also be done with the lower leg in *Padmasana*, when possible. It then works deep into the hip socket, pelvic ligaments and lower back, while challenging the *bandhas*. It releases the neck and strengthens the wrists. It promotes deep internalization and is extremely restful. The arms are used to support the back.

168

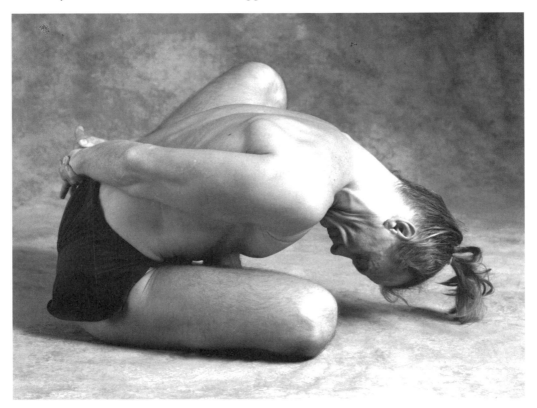

SUMMARY

Sit with both legs bent, one knee up (the 'up-knee'), one down (the 'down-knee'), with the up-knee heel against the down-knee ankle against the opposite buttock bone, and wrap its own arm round the upright shin and catch the other hand behind the waist. Press the up-knee foot down. Keeping the spine long, extend it forwards and down and relax the spine, shoulders and neck, keeping the feet and legs active. Maintain the *bandhas* with the abdomen long, hollow and empty, the chest broad and full, core of the body soft, with smooth, rhythmic *Ujjayi* breathing.

43

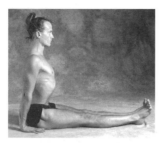

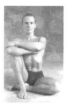

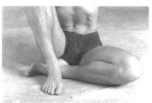

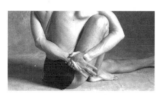

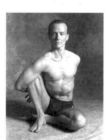

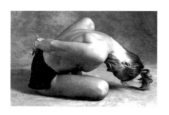

1 Sit on the floor with legs outstretched, straight and strong, feet together and alive, with your spine lifting straight out of your pelvis (*Dandasana*).

2 **Exhaling**, bend your legs so your left knee goes down and out with your heel against your right buttock bone, and your right heel comes against your left ankle with its foot flat and knee up. Catch hold of your right shin. Keep pressing your right foot firmly into the floor so the calf and thigh engage.

3 **Inhaling**, lift and broaden your ribcrest, sucking your solar plexus in and up so your chest becomes active, broad and full, your abdomen passive, long and empty (*Uddiyanabandha*) and flatten your pubic abdomen, with your anus soft as you suck your perineum and sacrum in (*Mulabandha*).

4 **Exhaling**, release your right hand and extend your right arm forward, while pulling low down on your right shin with your left hand.

5 **Inhaling**, lift and lengthen your spine.

6 **Exhaling**, lengthen your right arm and, keeping it straight and long, pull it back against your right shin so that your shin is in your armpit, not lower down your arm.

7 **Inhaling**, lift and lengthen your spine.

8 **Exhaling**, bend your right arm back around your shin to catch your left hand behind your waist.

9 **Inhaling**, lift and lengthen your spine.

10 **Exhaling**, extend your trunk forward inside your left knee, using your right arm against your shin bone as a lever to propel your spine forwards as you come down towards the leg. Relax your neck.

Hold with the left leg strong, right foot pressing the floor, neck, shoulders and spine relaxed, core of the body soft, *bandhas* engaged, with smooth, rhythmic *Ujjayi* breathing until ready to release back to *Dandasana* on an **inhalation**, maintaining the *bandhas*, and follow the breath through one of the short *vinyasa* sequences, and then repeat steps **2 to 10** on the other side. When you have done both sides, follow the breath through any of the *vinyasa* sequences to *Parivrttamarichyasana* (**43**). **43**

169

No. 43 Parivrttamarichyasana

Marichya Twist

This pose gives a gentle twist to your spine, softening the back muscles. It mobilizes the sacrum and sacroiliac joints, the spine, including the neck, stimulating blood flow to the spinal column. Preparation and counter-pose for backbends.

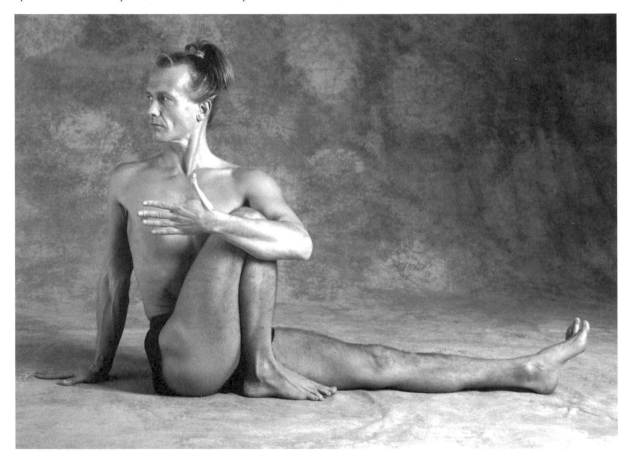

SUMMARY

Sitting with one leg straight, one bent with the foot in and knee up, wrap the straight leg arm round the upright shin and turn to look over the bent-leg shoulder. Keep the feet and legs alive, spine long, chest open, core of the body soft, maintaining the *bandhas* with the abdomen long, hollow and empty, the chest broad and full, with smooth, rhythmic *Ujjayi* breathing. 44 44

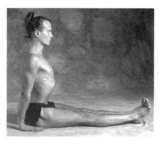

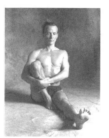

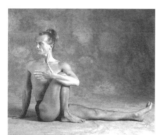

1 Sit on the floor with legs outstretched, straight and strong, feet together and alive, with your spine lifting straight out of your pelvis (*Dandasana*).

2 **Exhaling**, bend your right leg by drawing your foot into your pubis, keeping your knee straight up, and catch hold of your right shin with both hands.

3 **Inhaling**, lift and broaden your ribcrest, sucking your solar plexus in and up so your chest becomes active, broad and full, your abdomen passive, long and empty (*Uddiyanabandha*) and flatten your pubic abdomen, with your anus soft as you suck your perineum and sacrum in (*Mulabandha*), and raise the right arm long and straight.

4 **Exhaling**, pull on your shin with your left hand to keep it vertical while pressing your foot down, and turn to the right, taking your right hand around and down behind you. Press your right palm into the floor.

171

5 **Inhaling**, wrap your left elbow round your right shin and lift and lengthen your spine.

6 **Exhaling**, turn your head and look over your right shoulder.

Hold keeping feet and legs active, spine lifting, neck relaxed, chest open. Maintain the *bandhas* with your abdomen long, hollow and empty, your chest broad and full, core of the body soft with smooth, rhythmic *Ujjayi* breathing, until ready to release to *Dandasana* on an **inhalation**, then follow the breath through one of the short *vinyasa* sequences, and then repeat steps **2 to 6** on the other side. When you have done both sides, follow the breath through any of the *vinyasa* sequences to *Parivrttasukhamarichyasana* (**44**). **44** **44**

No. 44 Parivrttasukhamarichyasana

Easy Marichya Twist

This pose can also be done with the lower leg in *Padmasana*, when possible. It gives a gentle twist to your spine, softening the back muscles. It mobilizes the sacrum and sacroiliac joints, the spine, including the neck, stimulating blood flow to the spinal column. Preparation and counter-pose for backbends.

172

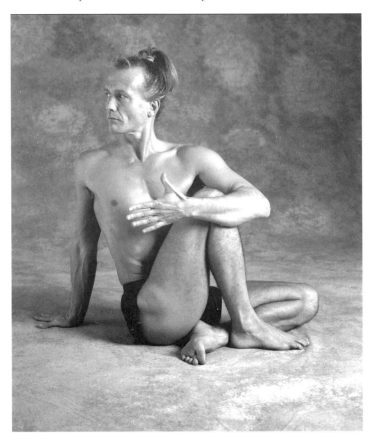

SUMMARY

With both legs bent, one knee up, one down, with the up-knee heel against the down-knee ankle against the upknee buttock bone, wrap the opposite arm round the upright shin and turn to look over that shoulder. Keep the upright knee foot active, spine long, chest open, core of the body soft, maintaining the *bandhas* with your abdomen long, hollow and empty, your chest broad and full, with smooth, rhythmic *Ujjayi* breathing. **47** **45**

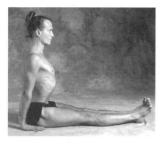

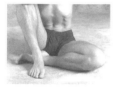

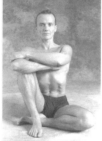

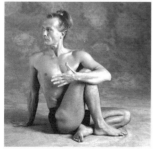

1 Sit on the floor with legs outstretched, straight and strong, feet together and alive, with your spine lifting straight out of your pelvis (*Dandasana*).

2 **Exhaling**, bend your legs so your left knee goes down and out with your heel against its buttock bone, and your right heel comes against your left ankle with its foot flat and knee up. Catch hold of your right shin with both hands.

3 **Inhaling**, lift and broaden your ribcrest, sucking your solar plexus in and up so your chest becomes active, broad and full, your abdomen passive, long and empty (*Uddiyanabandha*) and flatten your pubic abdomen, with your anus soft as you suck your perineum and sacrum in (*Mulabandha*), and raise your right arm long and straight.

4 **Exhaling**, pull on your shin with your left hand to keep it vertical while pressing your foot down and turn to the right taking your right hand around and down behind you. Press your right palm into the floor.

173

5 **Inhaling**, wrap your left elbow round your right shin and lift and lengthen your spine.

6 **Exhaling**, turn your head and look over your right shoulder.

Hold keeping right foot and leg active, spine lifting, neck relaxed, chest open. Maintain the *bandhas* with your abdomen long, hollow and empty, your chest broad and full, core of the body soft with smooth, rhythmic *Ujjayi* breathing, until ready to release to *Dandasana* on an **inhalation**, then follow the breath through one of the short *vinyasa* sequences, and then repeat steps **2 to 6** on the other side. When you have done both sides, follow the breath through any of the *vinyasa* sequences to the posture indicated below, for the Series you are practising.

47 **45**

No. 45 Dwihastabhujasana

The Pendulum

This pose must be done from the confidence of a quiet mind, and accurate weight placement, rather than brute force. If so, it becomes much easier than it may first appear. It develops strength in the hands, wrists and arms, develops balance and stability, and opens the lower back. It teaches the power of stillness in action.

174

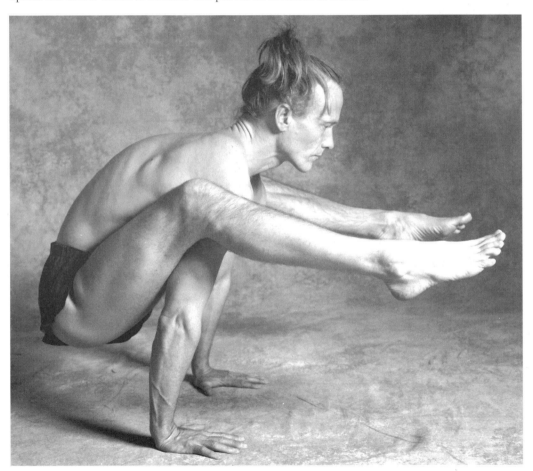

SUMMARY

From a squat, pass the arms through the backs of the legs, bringing the palms flat to the floor behind your feet. Lift the feet and balance all your weight on your palms. Maintain the *bandhas*, core of the body soft, with smooth, rhythmic *Ujjayi* breathing.

46

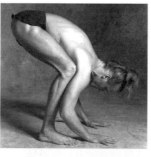

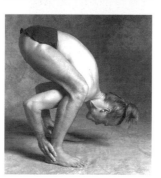

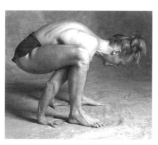

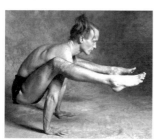

1 Stand with your feet hip-width apart and then bend your legs till you are squatting with your knees in your armpits, arms relaxed.

2 **Exhaling**, slip your arms through the backs of your legs, taking them as far through as possible. Use your hands on your ankles to gain some leverage to take the outer edge of your shoulder into the hollow of the back of your knee.

3 **Inhaling**, place your palms flat on the floor by your feet so that the edges of your heels lie inside the spaces between your thumbs and index fingers.

4 **Exhaling**, clarify the contact your hands have with the floor, keeping your palms broad, fingers centred and long as you press down firmly with the base of your index finger and the ball of your thumb.

175

5 **Inhaling**, lift and broaden your ribcrest, sucking your solar plexus in and up so your chest becomes active, broad and full, your abdomen passive, long and empty (*Uddiyanabandha*), and flatten your pubic abdomen, with your anus soft as you suck your perineum and sacrum in (*Mulabandha*).

6 **Exhaling**, lean your body weight back, full onto your hands, and lift your feet off the floor.

7 **Inhaling**, bring the balls of your big toes towards each other and straighten your arms as much as you can.

Hold, keeping your hands alive, allowing them to adjust their contact with the floor to absorb the movement of your body without losing your balance. Maintain the *bandhas* with your abdomen long, hollow and empty, your chest broad and full, core of your body soft, with smooth, rhythmic *Ujjayi* breathing. Release to *Dandasana*, then follow the breath through any of the *vinyasa* sequences to *Bakasana* (**46**). **46**

No. 46 Bakasana

The Crow Pose

This pose must be done from the confidence of a quiet mind, and accurate use of hands and arms, rather than sheer strength. If so, it becomes much easier than it may first appear. It not only develops poise and balance while strengthening the arms but, in its full form, with the knees deep in the armpits, gives a deep, satisfying stretch to the lower back.

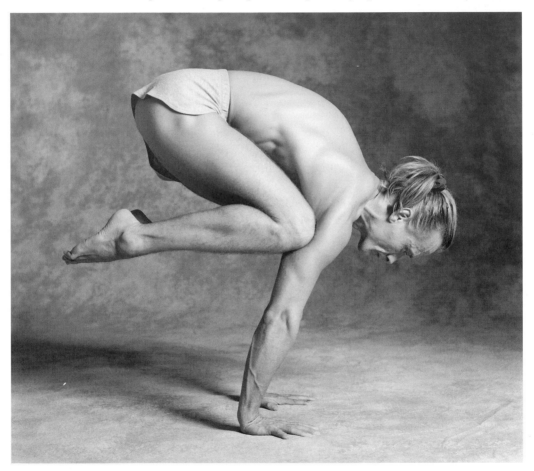

SUMMARY
From a squat balance, on your hands with your knees deep in your armpits and your arms straight. Maintain the *bandhas*, core of the body soft, with smooth, rhythmic *Ujjayi* breathing. **48**

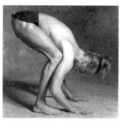

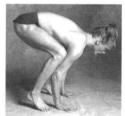

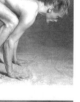

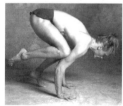

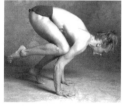

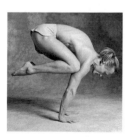

1   Stand with your feet hip-width apart and then bend your legs till you are squatting with your knees in your armpits, arms relaxed.

2   Bring your palms flat to the floor in line with but in front of your feet.

3   **Exhaling**, bring your weight forwards onto your palms, pressing your shinbones into your upper arms as you lift your heels as high as you can keeping the weight mostly on your hands and some on the balls of your feet.

4   **Inhaling**, lift and broaden your ribcrest, sucking your solar plexus in and up so your chest becomes active, broad and full, your abdomen passive, long and empty (*Uddiyanabandha*), and flatten your pubic abdomen, with your anus soft as you suck your perineum and sacrum in (*Mulabandha*).

5   **Exhaling**, carefully lift one foot as high off the floor as you can.

6   **Inhaling**, establish your stability.

7   **Exhaling**, carefully lift your second foot as high off the floor as you can.

8   **Inhaling**, pull your knees deep into your armpits and straighten your arms.

Hold, keeping your hands alive, allowing them to adjust their contact with the floor to absorb the movement of your body without losing your balance. Maintain the *bandhas* with your abdomen long, hollow and empty, your chest broad and full, core of your body soft, with smooth, rhythmic *Ujjayi* breathing. Release to *Dandasana*, then follow the breath through any of the *vinyasa* sequences to *Baddhakonasana* (**48**). **48**

177

No. 47 Urdhvabaddhakonasana

The Cobbler

This pose is the traditional seat of the Indian cobbler. Do not force the knees down, they will go down when the hips open. It opens the hip joints, stretches the inner thighs, mobilizes the ankles and the knees. It clarifies the use of the *bandhas* to elevate the spine. Preparation for *Baddhakonasana* and *Padmasana*.

178

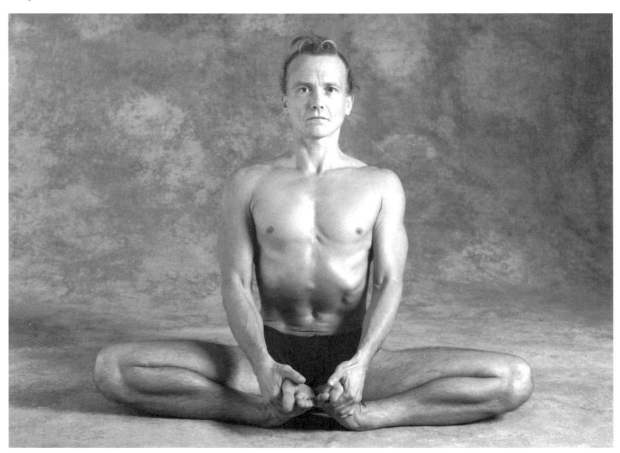

SUMMARY

Sit with the feet together in front of you, using your fingers and thumbs to open them like a book and use the grip of your hands and your arms to lengthen the spine. Clarify the *bandhas* with the abdomen long, hollow and empty, the chest broad and full, and soften the core of the body with smooth, rhythmic *Ujjayi* breathing. 52 **50**

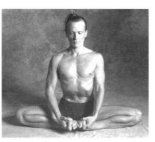

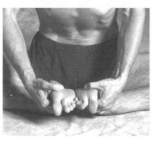

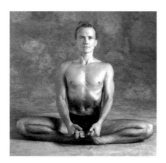

1   Sit on the floor with your feet and legs relaxed in front of you.

2   Take hold of each foot in its own hand so that the tops of your feet are resting in the insides of your hands with your thumbs round the bottom of the balls of your big toes, your fingers gripping the outer edge of your foot.

3   **Exhaling**, slip the balls of your thumbs onto the balls of your big toes and, pressing hard with them, push the inner edges of your feet out and away from each other as you use the fingers on the bone of the outer edge of your foot to push them in and up towards you so that your feet open like a book with the soles showing. To the extent that your ankles are mobile and your feet open, your knees will go down naturally. Do not force them down.

4   **Inhaling**, lift and broaden your ribcrest, sucking your solar plexus in and up so your chest becomes active, broad and full, your abdomen passive, long and empty (*Uddiyanabandha*), and flatten your pubic abdomen, with your anus soft as you suck your perineum and sacrum in (*Mulabandha*). Your waist and spine should lengthen considerably. Use your hands and arms as levers to enhance this effect.

5   **Exhaling**, use your hands and arms as levers to lengthen your waist, lift your spine and open your chest, while pressing the soles of your feet together and drawing the inner thighs out of your pelvis.

Hold while working your feet to open more, clarify the *bandhas* and soften the core of your body with smooth, rhythmic *Ujjayi* breathing, till ready to release into one of the breath-determined *vinyasa* sequences to the posture indicated below for the Series you are practising. ✦ 50

179

No. 48 Baddhakonasana

Resting Cobbler Pose

This pose develops flexibility in the hips, knees and ankles. Great care must be taken not to strain the lower back by forcing the head down. Preparation for *Padmasana*.

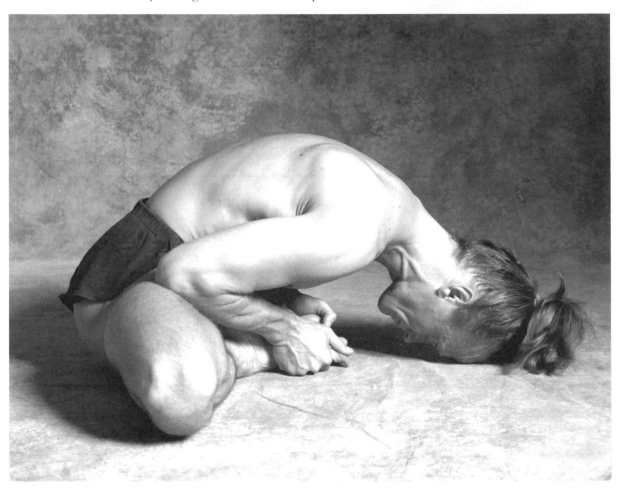

SUMMARY

Sit with the feet together in front of you, using your fingers and thumbs to open them like a book and use the grip of your hands and your arms to lengthen the spine. Bring the trunk forward and down, head towards the floor. Clarify the *bandhas* and soften the core of the body with smooth, rhythmic *Ujjayi* breathing.

49

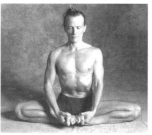

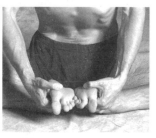

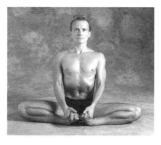

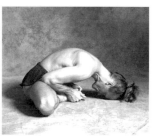

1   Sit on the floor with your feet and legs relaxed and bent in front of you.

2   Take hold of each foot in its own hand so that the tops of your feet are resting in the insides of your hands with your thumbs round the bottom of the balls of your big toes, your fingers gripping the outer edge of your foot.

3   **Exhaling**, slip the balls of your thumbs onto the balls of your big toes and, pressing hard with them, push the inner edges of your feet down and away from each other as you use the fingers on the bone of the outer edge of your foot to push them towards each other so that your feet open like a book with the soles showing. To the extent that your ankles are mobile and your feet open, your knees will go down naturally. Do not force them down.

4   **Inhaling**, lift and broaden your ribcrest, sucking your solar plexus in and up so your chest becomes active, broad and full, your abdomen passive, long and empty (*Uddiyanabandha*), and flatten your pubic abdomen, with your anus soft as you suck your perineum and sacrum in (*Mulabandha*). Your waist and spine should lengthen considerably. Use the hands and arms as levers to enhance this effect, while pressing the soles of your feet together and drawing the inner thighs out of your pelvis. (*Urdhvabaddhakonasana* hold here a while if you have not already done this pose.)

181

5   **Exhaling**, slowly pivot your pelvis, rolling your hip bones forward, and extend your trunk forward and down towards the floor. Relax your neck towards the floor. Take care not to force your way down.

Hold while working the feet to open more, keep your waist as long as you can, clarify the *bandhas* and so ten the core of your body with smooth, rhythmic *Ujjayi* breathing, till ready to release to *Dandasana*, then follow the breath through any of the *vinyasa* sequences to *Merudandasana* (**49**), or go straight from holding step **5** into steps **3 to 6** of *Merudandasana* (**49**) without a *vinyasa*.

No. 49 Merudandasana

Wide Balancing Pose

This pose opens the hips and tones the legs while developing poise, balance and quietness of mind. It teaches the relationship between the activity of the legs, the *bandhas* and elevation of the spine. In the Preparatory Series it can be done as a direct continuation of *Baddhakonasana*, and/or immediately before *Upavistakonasana* without a connecting *vinyasa*.

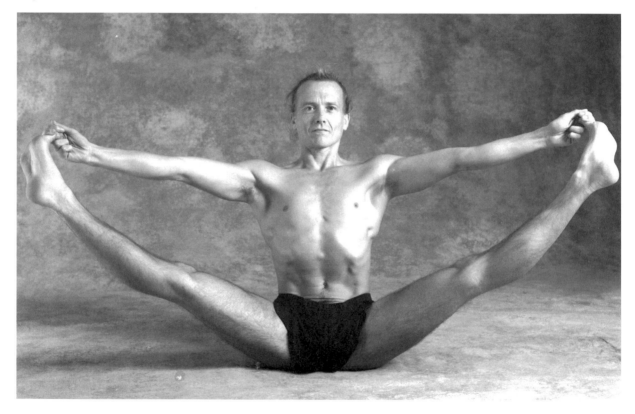

SUMMARY

Balance on the buttock bones with the legs straight and wide apart holding the big toes. Maintain the *bandhas* with the abdomen long, hollow and empty, the chest broad and full, and soften the core of the body with smooth, rhythmic *Ujjayi* breathing.

51

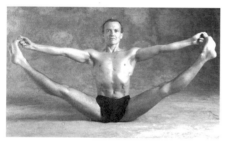

1 Sit on the floor with your feet and legs relaxed in front of you.

2 Bend your legs and take hold of each of your big toes in the thumbs and first two fingers of their respective hands.

3 Lifting your feet off the floor, balance on your buttocks with your legs still bent.

4 **Inhaling**, lift and broaden your ribcrest, sucking your solar plexus in and up so your chest becomes active, broad and full, your abdomen passive, long and empty (*Uddiyanabandha*), and flatten your pubic abdomen, with your anus soft as you suck your perineum and sacrum in (*Mulabandha*).

5 **Exhaling**, take your feet away from each other and your trunk, straightening your legs as much as possible.

6 **Inhaling**, use your hands and arms as levers against your legs and lengthen your waist, spine and neck, looking forwards.

183

Hold with legs straight and strong, arms long, clarify the *bandhas* and soften the core of your body with smooth, rhythmic *Ujjayi* breathing, till ready to release to *Dandasana*, then follow the breath through any of the *vinyasa* sequences to *Upavistakonasana* (**51**), or **exhale** from holding step **6** straight into *Upavistakonasana* (**51**) step **5**, without a *vinyasa*. **51**

No. 50 Urdhvakonasana

Sitting Splits Pose

This pose gives a gentle stretch to the inner thigh muscles, tones the legs, awakens the feet and opens the hips. It teaches the relationship between the quality of the feet and the activity of the legs. Preparation for *Upavistakonasana*.

184

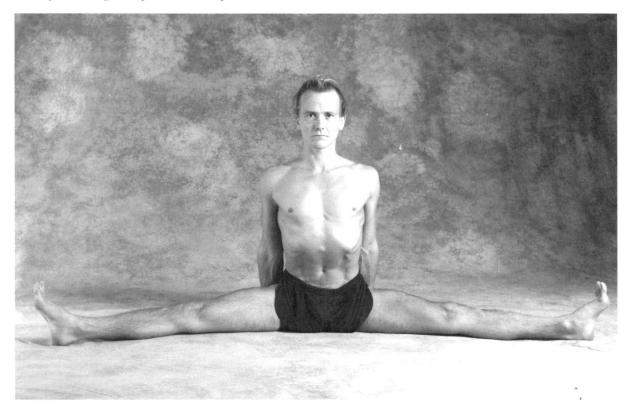

SUMMARY

Sit with legs spread wide apart and strong, lifting the spine up out of the pelvis. Maintain the *bandhas* with the abdomen long, hollow and empty, the chest broad and full, core of the body soft, with smooth, rhythmic *Ujjayi* breathing. **52**

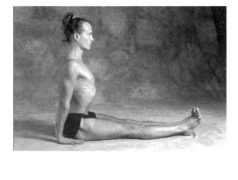

1 Sit on the floor with legs outstretched, straight and strong, feet together and alive, with your spine lifting straight out of your pelvis (*Dandasana*).

2 **Exhaling**, take your feet wide apart, spreading your legs as much as possible.

3 **Inhaling**, place your hands on the floor behind your buttocks and, lifting them a fraction, push your pelvis forwards to spread your legs further.

4 **Exhaling**, extend your legs, broadening the ball of your foot, lengthening the inner heel and front ankle and sucking your thigh muscles in so the backs of your knees go down as your legs straighten.

5 **Inhaling**, lift and broaden your ribcrest, sucking your solar plexus in and up so your chest becomes active, broad and full, your abdomen passive, long and empty (*Uddiyanabandha*), and flatten your pubic abdomen, with your anus soft as you suck your perineum and sacrum in (*Mulabandha*).

185

6 **Exhaling**, press your palms firmly into the floor behind your buttocks and, lengthening your waist, lift your spine and open your chest.

Hold, keeping legs strong, feet alive, maintaining the *bandhas*, core of your body soft, with smooth, rhythmic *Ujjayi* breathing, till ready to release to *Dandasana*, then follow the breath through any of the *vinyasa* sequences to *Supturdhvapadangus-tasana* (**52**).

52

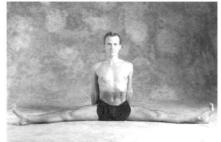

No. 51 Upavistakonasana

Bowing Splits Pose

This pose can be done as a continuation of *Merudandasana*. It gives an intense stretch to the inner thigh muscles, tones the legs, awakens the feet and releases the hips, while stretching the back. It teaches the relationship between the quality of the feet and the activity of the legs.

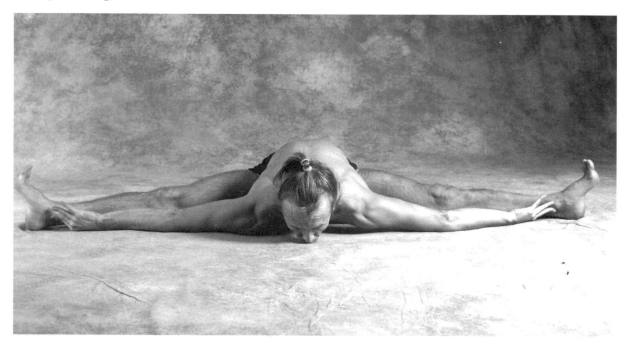

SUMMARY

Sit with legs spread wide apart and bring the trunk forwards along the floor in front of you. Maintain the *bandhas* with the abdomen long, hollow and empty, the chest broad and full, core of the body soft, with smooth, rhythmic *Ujjayi* breathing. **52**

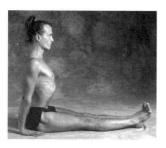

1 Sit on the floor with legs outstretched, straight and strong, feet together and alive, with your spine lifting straight out of your pelvis (*Dandasana*).

2 **Exhaling**, take your feet wide apart, spreading your legs as much as possible.

3 **Inhaling**, place your hands on the floor behind your buttocks and, lifting them a fraction, push your pelvis forwards to spread your legs further.

4 **Exhaling**, extend your legs, broadening the ball of your foot, lengthening the inner heel and front ankle and sucking your thigh muscles in so the backs of your knees go down as your legs straighten.

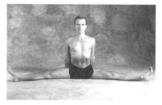

5 **Inhaling**, lift and broaden your ribcrest, sucking your solar plexus in and up so your chest becomes active, broad and full, your abdomen passive, long and empty (*Uddiyanabandha*), and flatten your pubic abdomen, with your anus soft as you suck your perineum and sacrum in (*Mulabandha*). (*Urdhvakonasana* hold here a while before continuing if you have not already done this pose.)

187

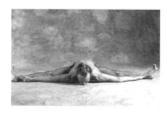

6 **Exhaling**, pivot your pelvis, rolling your hipbones forwards, and extend your trunk forward and down towards the floor. Use your hands like sucker pads in front of you, step by step, to draw you forwards and down. Relax your neck towards the floor, and take your hands to your ankles. Take care not to force your way down.

Hold, keeping legs strong and centred, feet alive, maintaining the *bandhas*, core of your body soft, with smooth, rhythmic *Ujjayi* breathing, till ready to release to *Dandasana*, then follow the breath through one of the *vinyasa* sequences to *Supturdhvapadangustasana* (**52**). **52**

No. 52 Supturdhvapadangustasana

Lying Triangle Pose

This pose rests the body while straightening and toning the legs. It clarifies the action of *Uddiyanabandha*. Preparation for *Suptaparsvapadangustasana*.

188

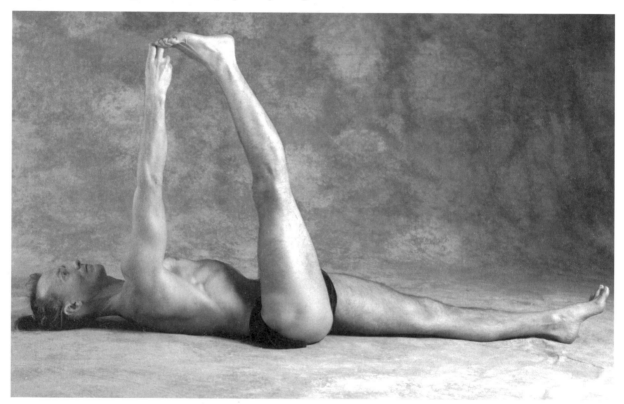

SUMMARY

Lying on your back with both legs long and strong, raise and straighten one leg, holding its big toe, keeping the feet alive. Maintain the *bandhas* with the abdomen long, hollow and empty, the chest broad and full, core of the body soft with smooth, rhythmic *Ujjayi* breathing.

⭐11 53 53

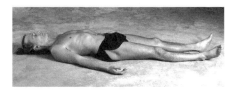

1 Lie flat on your back in *Savasana*.

2 **Exhaling**, suck your thigh muscles into your legs and, broadening the balls of your feet, engage your calf muscles. At the same time, lengthen the front and inner ankle and the Achilles tendon, so your foot is alive and your ankle joint evenly open.

3 **Inhaling**, broaden your ribcrest and suck your solar plexus in and up so your chest becomes active, broad and full, your abdomen passive, long and empty (*Uddiyanabandha*), and flatten your pubic abdomen, sucking your perineum in with your anus soft (*Mulabandha*).

4 **Exhaling**, bend your right leg and lift your knee towards you, keeping your left leg active, straight, long and strong.

5 **Inhaling**, catch your big toe with your right thumb and first two fingers.

189

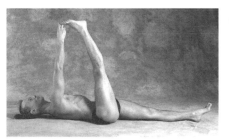

6 **Exhaling**, use the grip of your right hand and straighten your right leg while at the same time lengthening and straightening your right arm and rolling its shoulder away from your leg towards the floor. Keep your left leg straight and strong, shoulders and head on the floor while looking at your right foot.

Hold with both legs straight, long and strong, feet alive, right arm long and straight, Maintain the *bandhas* with the abdomen long, hollow and empty, the chest broad and full, core of your body soft with smooth, rhythmic *Ujjayi* breathing till ready to release to *Savasana*, and then change legs and repeat steps **2 to 6** on the other side. Roll back to *Dandasana* when you have done both sides, then follow the breath through one of the *vinyasa* sequences to the posture indicated below, for the Series you are practising. ✦ 11 53 53

No. 53 Suptaparsvapadangustasana

Lying Side Triangle Pose

This pose rests the body while opening the hips and straightening and toning the legs. It clarifies the action of *Uddiyanabandha*. It is usually done as a continuation of *Suptapadangustasana*.

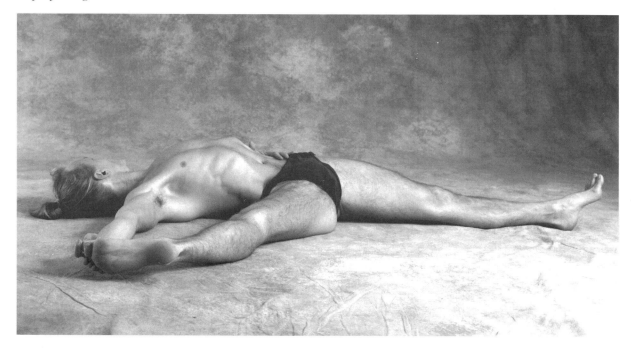

SUMMARY

Lying on your back with both legs long and strong, extend and straighten one leg out to the side and towards the floor, holding its big toe, keeping the feet alive, while looking to the other side. Maintain the *bandhas*, abdomen long hollow and empty, chest broad and full, core of the body soft with smooth, rhythmic *Ujjayi* breathing. **55** **54**

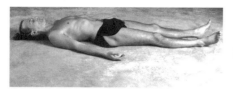

1 Lie flat on your back in *Savasana*.

2 **Exhaling**, suck the thigh muscles into your legs and, broadening the balls of your feet, engage your calf muscles. At the same time, lengthen the front and inner ankle and the Achilles tendon, so your foot is alive and your ankle joint evenly open.

3 **Inhaling**, broaden your ribcrest and suck your solar plexus in and up so your chest becomes active, broad and full, your abdomen passive, long and empty (*Uddiyanabandha*), and flatten your pubic abdomen, sucking your perineum in with your anus soft (*Mulabandha*).

4 **Exhaling**, bend your right leg and lift the knee towards you, keeping your left leg active, straight, long and strong.

5 **Inhaling**, catch the big toe with your right thumb and first two fingers.

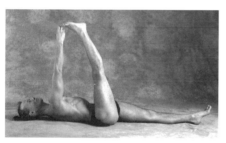

6 **Exhaling**, use the grip of your right hand and straighten your right leg while at the same time lengthening and straightening your right arm and rolling its shoulder away from your leg towards the floor. (*Suptapadangustasana* (**52**), hold here a while before continuing if you have not already done this pose.)

7 **Inhaling**, and keeping your left thigh, buttock, hip and lower back down, take your right leg out and down towards the floor. Turn and look the other way, keeping your left leg strong and straight, head and shoulders on the floor. Do not force your leg to the floor if the left side of your body rises, or the pose will not work to open the hip.

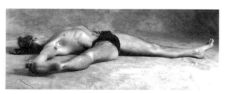

Hold with both legs straight, long and strong, feet alive, right arm long and straight, maintain the *bandhas* with the abdomen long, hollow and empty, the chest broad and full, core of your body soft with smooth, rhythmic *Ujjayi* breathing, until ready to release to *Savasana*, and then repeat steps **2 to 7** on the other side. Roll back to *Dandasana* when you have done both sides, then follow the breath through one of the *vinyasa* sequences to the next posture indicated below, for the Series you are practising.

55 **54**

191

No. 54 Ubbayapadangustasana

Toe Balancing Pose

This pose develops balance while straightening and toning the legs. It teaches the relationship between straight legs, the *bandhas* and spinal elevation. Preparation for *Navasana*. It can be done in a single flowing sequence of *Ubbayapadangustasana* (**54**), *Navasana* (**56**), *Ubbayapadhastasana* (**57**), *Navasana* (**56**), *Pascimottanasana* (**58**) without connecting *vinyasas*.

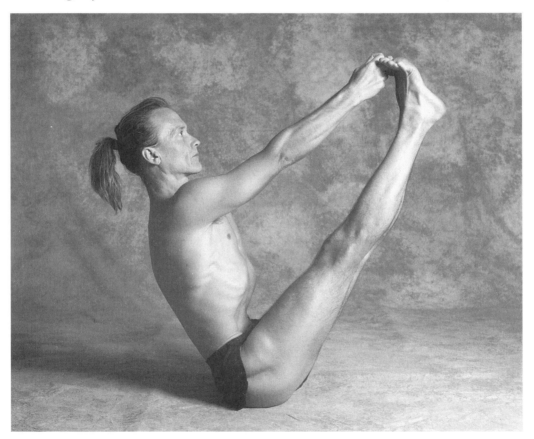

SUMMARY

Balance on your buttocks, legs straight and together holding the big toes, with the feet alive. Keep the spine long, chest open, maintaining the *bandhas* with the abdomen long, hollow and empty, the chest broad and full, core of the body soft, with smooth, rhythmic *Ujjayi* breathing. **56**

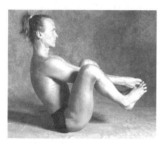

1 Sit on the floor with legs outstretched, straight and strong, feet together and alive, with your spine lifting straight out of your pelvis (*Dandasana*).

2 Relax your legs, bend them and catch hold of the big toes of each foot.

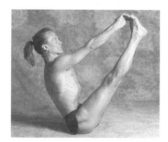

3 **Inhaling**, roll back a little so you are balancing on your buttocks, feet off the ground.

4 **Exhaling**, take your feet away from your trunk so that your legs straighten as much as possible, and look towards your feet. To straighten your legs you may need to slide your hands down on to your shins.

193

5 **Inhaling**, lift and broaden your ribcrest, sucking your solar plexus in and up so your chest becomes active, broad and full, your abdomen passive, long and empty (*Uddiyanabandha*), and flatten your pubic abdomen, with your anus soft as you suck your perineum and sacrum in (*Mulabandha*).

Hold with your legs straight and strong, your feet alive, your spine long, chest open and smooth rhythmic *Ujjayi* breathing, until ready to release to *Dandasana* on an **inhalation**, then follow the breath through one of the *vinyasa* sequences to the next posture *Navasana* (**56**), which you may flow directly into step **5** of without a connecting *vinyasa*.

56

No. 55 Sukhanavasana

Easy Boat Pose

This pose develops balance while straightening and toning the legs. It teaches the relationship between the actions of legs, *bandhas* and spine. Preparation for *Navasana*.

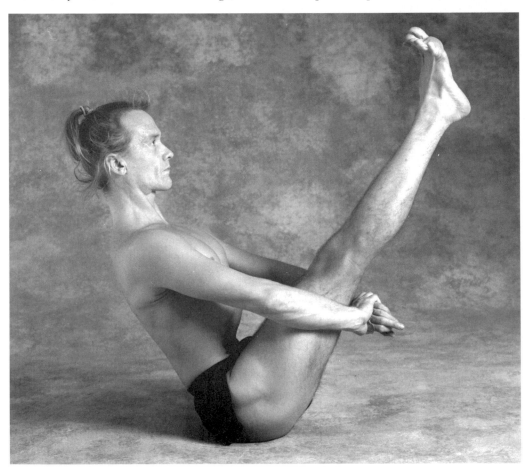

SUMMARY

Balance on your buttocks, legs straight and together forming a V with your trunk, while supporting the legs with your arms clasped behind the backs of the knees, feet alive. Keep the spine long, chest open, maintaining the *bandhas* with the abdomen long, hollow and empty, the chest broad and full, core of your body soft, with smooth, rhythmic *Ujjayi* breathing.

59

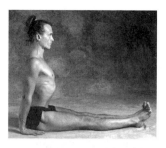

1 Sit on the floor with legs outstretched, straight and strong, feet together and alive, with your spine lifting straight out of your pelvis (*Dandasana*).

2 Relax your legs and draw your feet in, knees up, and pass your arms through the backs of your knees, holding one hand or wrist with the other.

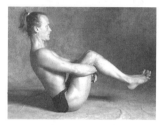

3 **Inhaling**, roll back a little so you are balancing on your buttocks, feet off the ground.

4 **Exhaling**, straighten your legs against the resistance of your held hands, and look ahead.

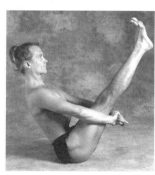

5 **Inhaling**, lift and broaden your ribcrest, sucking your solar plexus in and up so your chest becomes active, broad and full, your abdomen passive, long and empty (*Uddiyanabandha*), and flatten your pubic abdomen, with your anus soft as you suck your perineum and sacrum in (*Mulabandha*).

Hold with the legs straight and strong, feet alive, the spine long, chest open and smooth rhythmic *Ujjayi* breathing, until ready to release to *Dandasana* on an **inhalation**, then follow the breath through one of the *vinyasa* sequences to *Ardhapurvot-tanasana* (**59**).

59

195

No. 56 Navasana

Boat Pose

This pose develops the back and thigh muscles, and develops balance. This is one of the most difficult poses in which to establish the *bandhas*. Care must be taken not to tighten the abdomen and shorten the spine. It can be done in a single flowing sequence of *Ubbayapadangustasana* (**54**), *Navasana* (**56**), *Ubbayapadhastasana* (**57**), *Navasana* (**56**), *Pascimottanasana* (**58**) without connecting *vinyasas*.

196

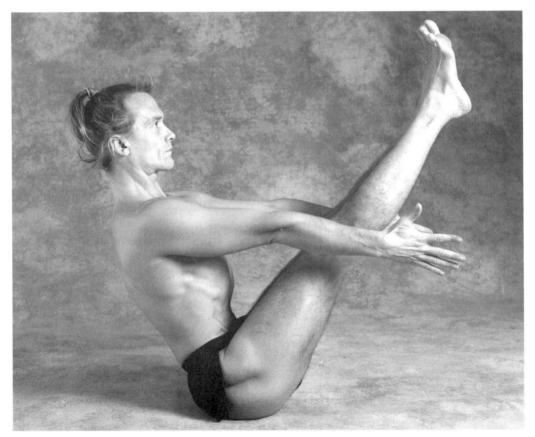

SUMMARY
Balance on your buttocks, legs raised straight and together so they form a V with your trunk, feet alive, arms parallel to the floor. Keep the spine long, chest open, maintaining the *bandhas* with the abdomen long, hollow and empty, the chest broad and full, core of your body soft, with smooth, rhythmic *Ujjayi* breathing. **57** **58**

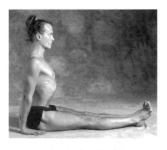

1   Sit on the floor with legs outstretched, straight and strong, feet together and alive, with your spine lifting straight out of your pelvis (*Dandasana*).

2   Relax your legs and draw your feet in, knees up.

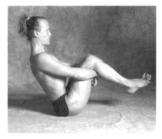

3   **Inhaling**, roll back a little so you are balancing on your buttocks, feet off the ground.

4   **Exhaling**, straighten your legs directly in front of you, keeping them together, keeping your abdomen hollow and passive, and extend your arms parallel to the floor, looking ahead through your legs.

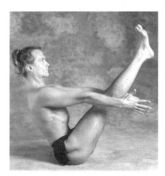

5   **Inhaling**, lift and broaden your ribcrest, sucking your solar plexus in and up so your chest becomes active, broad and full, your abdomen passive, long and empty (*Uddiyanabandha*), and flatten your pubic abdomen, with your anus soft as you suck your perineum and sacrum in (*Mulabandha*).

Hold with your legs straight and strong, feet alive, your spine long, chest open and smooth rhythmic *Ujjayi* breathing, until ready to release to *Dandasana* on an **exhalation**, then follow the breath through one of the *vinyasa* sequences to *Ubbayapadahastasana* (**57**) or flow directly into it without a *vinyasa* by catching the heels. **57** **58**

197

No. 57 Ubbayapadahastasana

Heel Balancing Pose

This pose develops balance while straightening and toning the legs. It teaches the relationship between the actions of legs, *bandhas* and spine. Preparation for *Navasana*. It can be done in a single flowing sequence of *Ubbayapadangustasana* (**54**), *Navasana* (**56**), *Ubbayapadahastasana* (**57**), *Navasana* (**56**), *Pascimottanasana* (**58**) without connecting *vinyasas*.

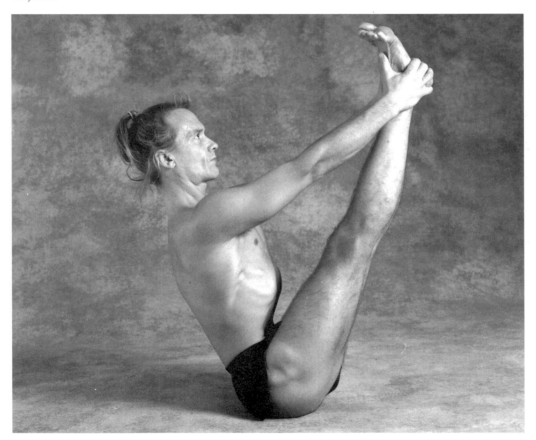

SUMMARY
Balance on your buttocks, legs straight and together, holding the heels with the feet alive. Keep the spine long, chest open, maintaining the *bandhas* with the abdomen long, hollow and empty, the chest broad and full, core of your body soft, with smooth, rhythmic *Ujjayi* breathing. **56** or **58**

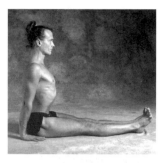

1 Sit on the floor with legs outstretched, straight and strong, feet together and alive, with your spine lifting straight out of your pelvis (*Dandasana*).

2 Relax your legs, bend them and catch hold of the heels of each foot.

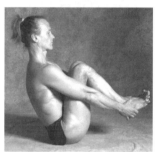

3 **Inhaling**, roll back a little so you are balancing on your buttocks, feet off the ground.

4 **Exhaling**, take your feet away from your trunk so that your legs straighten as much as possible, keeping them together. Look to your feet. To straighten your legs you may need to slide your hands down on to your shins.

199

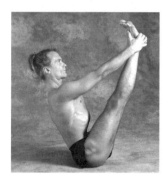

5 **Inhaling**, lift and broaden your ribcrest, sucking your solar plexus in and up so your chest becomes active, broad and full, your abdomen passive, long and empty (*Uddiyanabandha*), and flatten your pubic abdomen, with your anus soft as you suck your perineum and sacrum in (*Mulabandha*).

Hold with your legs straight and strong, feet alive, your spine long, chest open and smooth rhythmic *Ujjayi* breathing, until ready to release to *Dandasana* on an **exhalation**, then follow the breath through one of the *vinyasa* sequences to *Pascimottanasana* (**58**), or flow into it via a few breaths in *Navasana* (**56**). **56** or **58**

No. 58 Pascimottanasana

Closed Vice Pose

This pose straightens and tones the legs, awakens the feet, releases the spine and promotes internalization. It teaches the effect of the *bandhas* on the spine and the importance of charging the legs and feet. It can be done in a single flowing sequence of *Ubbayapadangustasana* (**54**), *Navasana* (**56**), *Ubbayapadhastasana* (**57**), *Navasana* (**56**), *Pascimottanasana* (**58**) without connecting *vinyasas*.

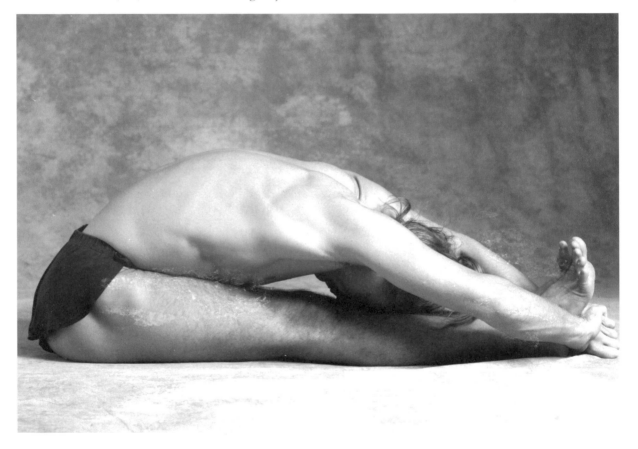

SUMMARY

With legs straight and feet alive, extend the spine forwards and down along the straight leg. Relaxing the spine and neck, charge the legs and feet. Core of the body soft, maintain the *bandhas* with the abdomen long, hollow and empty, the chest broad and full with smooth, rhythmic *Ujjayi* breathing.

60

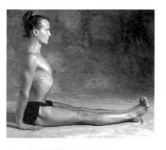

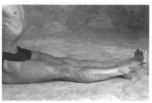

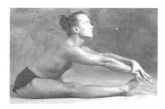

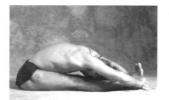

1   Sit on the floor with legs outstretched, straight and strong, feet together and alive, with your spine lifting straight out of your pelvis (*Dandasana*).

2   **Exhaling**, extend your legs, broadening the ball of your foot, lengthening your inner heel and front ankle and sucking your thigh muscles in so the backs of your knees go down as your legs straighten.

3   **Inhaling**, lift and broaden your ribcrest, sucking your solar plexus in and up so your chest becomes active, broad and full, your abdomen passive, long and empty (*Uddiyanabandha*), and flatten your pubic abdomen, with your anus soft as you suck your perineum and sacrum in (*Mulabandha*).

4   **Exhaling**, pivot your pelvis and reach forward with both hands and catch your shin, ankle or foot of each leg, keeping them straight, your feet alive.

5   **Inhaling**, clarify the *bandhas* as you lift your chin, lengthen the front of your spine and open your chest, keeping your legs straight.

6   **Exhaling**, bend your arms, drawing your elbows forward, and lengthen the front of your spine forwards as it comes down towards your legs, and relax your neck. Keep your legs straight.

7   **Inhaling**, clarify the *bandhas* as you draw your chin forward, lengthen the front of your spine and open your chest, keeping your legs straight.

Hold, with your legs strong, feet alive, core of your body soft, maintaining the *bandhas* with smooth, rhythmic *Ujjayi* breathing, till ready to release by **Inhaling**, to *Dandasana*, while maintaining the charge in your legs and trunk, then follow the breath through one of the *vinyasa* sequences to *Purvottanasana* (**60**).

60

201

No. 59 Ardhapurvottanasana

Half Opening Pose

This pose stretches and tones the front of the torso, and develops the arms, and wrists. It is a mild counter-pose to *Pascimottanasana* cycle. It is a preparation for *Purvottanasana*.

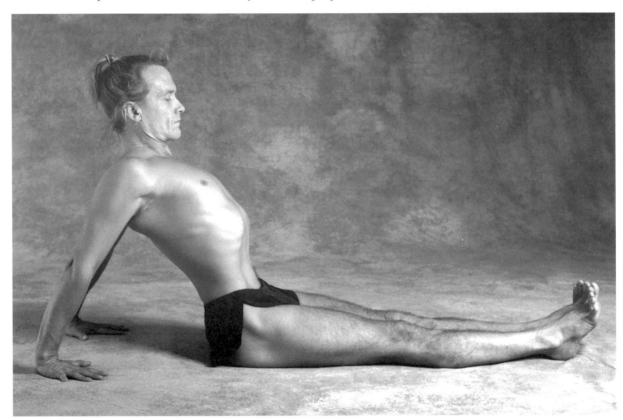

SUMMARY

Sitting with legs in front, straight and strong, feet alive, lean back onto your palms and lift and open your chest. Maintain the *bandhas* with the abdomen long, hollow and empty, the chest broad and full, core of the body soft, with smooth, rhythmic *Ujjayi* breathing.

13

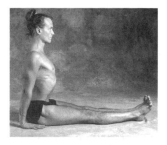

1 Sit on the floor with legs outstretched, straight and strong, feet together and alive, with your spine lifting straight out of your pelvis (*Dandasana*).

2 **Inhaling**, lean back and place your hands behind you, palms down, fingers pointing towards you.

3 **Exhaling**, engage your palms against the floor and straighten your arms, broadening the base of your fingers, lengthening your fingers and pressing the base of your index finger firmly into the floor. Keep your legs strong, sucking your thigh muscles in, feet alive.

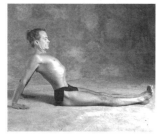

4 **Inhaling**, gently arching your back, lift and broaden your ribcrest, sucking your solar plexus in and up so your chest becomes active, broad and full, your abdomen passive, long and empty (*Uddiyanabandha*), and flatten your pubic abdomen, with your anus soft as you suck your perineum and sacrum in (*Mulabandha*).

203

Hold, looking towards your toes, keeping the abdomen long, empty and hollow, the chest high, broad and full with your legs strong and feet alive. When ready, release to *Dandasana*, and follow the breath through one of the *vinyasa* sequences to *Ardhurdhvamukhasvanasana* (**13**).

13

No. 6o Purvottanasana

Opening Pose

This pose stretches and tones the front of the legs and torso, develops the arms, strengthens the wrists and releases and strengthens the ankles. It is a counter-pose to *Pascimottanasana* cycle.

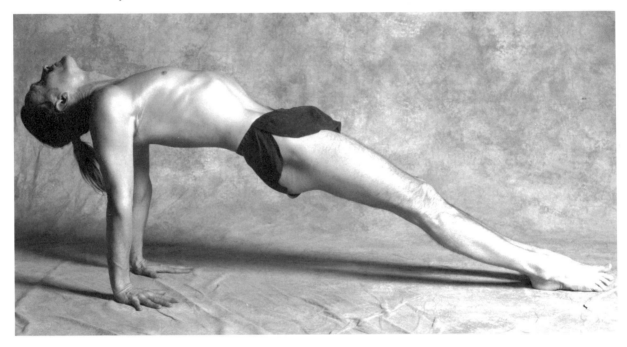

SUMMARY

Sitting with legs in front, straight and strong, lean back onto your palms and lift and open your chest, and lift the pelvis off the floor so that the soles of the feet come down to the floor. Maintain the *bandhas* with the abdomen long, hollow and empty, the chest broad and full, core of the body soft, with smooth, rhythmic *Ujjayi* breathing. **64**

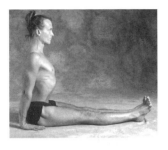

1 Sit on the floor with legs outstretched, straight and strong, feet together and alive, with your spine lifting straight out of your pelvis (*Dandasana*).

2 **Inhaling**, lean back and place your hands behind you, palms down, fingers pointing towards you.

3 **Exhaling**, engage your palms against the floor and straighten your arms, broadening the base of your fingers, lengthening your fingers and pressing the base of your index finger firmly into the floor. Keep your legs strong, sucking your thigh muscles in, feet alive.

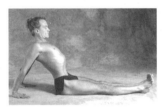

4 **Inhaling**, lift and broaden your ribcrest, sucking your solar plexus in and up so your chest becomes active, broad and full, your abdomen passive, long and empty (*Uddiyanabandha*), and flatten your pubic abdomen, with your anus soft as you suck your perineum and sacrum in (*Mulabandha*). (*Ardhapurvottanasana;* hold here a while if you have not already done this pose.)

205

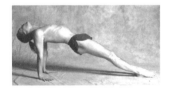

5 **Exhaling**, raise your buttocks off the floor as high as you can, keeping your legs straight and strong, and bring the soles of your feet onto the floor.

6 **Inhaling**, take your head back by taking your chin up and back in a wide arc while taking the base of your skull forward, in and up.

Hold, keeping your abdomen long, empty and hollow, your chest high, broad and full with your legs strong and feet alive. When ready, release to *Dandasana*, then follow the breath through one of the *vinyasa* sequences to *Ardhapindasana* (**64**). **64**

No. 61 Setubhujasana

Shoulder Bridge Pose

This pose is a backbend and can therefore trouble the lumbar spine (lower back) if not approached with care. The key is correct use of the feet, keeping the back muscles soft, using the *bandhas* and activating the full length of the spine. It tones the front of the body, lengthens the front thighs and opens the chest.

206

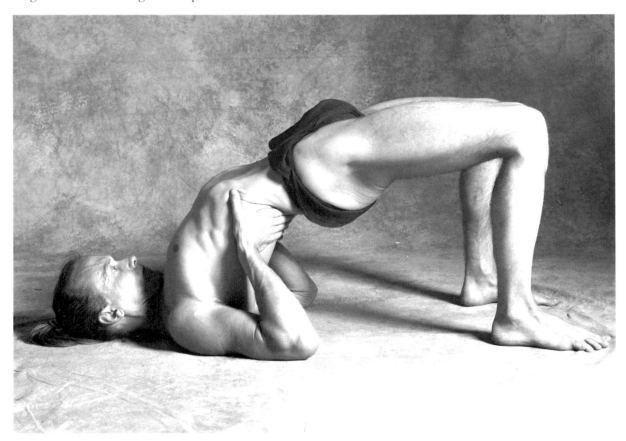

SUMMARY

Lying on your back, tuck your feet in keeping them stable, even and alive and, keeping the shoulders and head down, raise the pelvis and arch the back, bring the palms under for support as you lift your spine as deeply in towards the front of your body as you can. Keep the feet strong, maintain the *bandhas*, with your ribcrest broad, chest broad and full, with smooth, rhythmic *Ujjayi* breathing, core of the body soft. **64** **62**

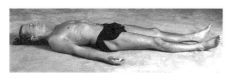

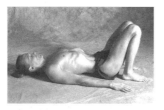

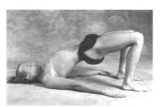

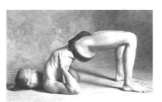

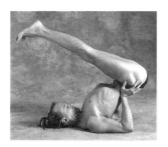

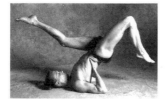

1   Lie in *Savasana*.

2   **Exhaling**, draw your heels in towards your buttocks, keeping your feet parallel, heels in line with your buttock bones.

3   **Inhaling**, broaden your ribcrest and suck your solar plexus in and up so your chest becomes active, broad and full, your abdomen passive, long and empty (*Uddiyanabandha*), and flatten your pubic abdomen, sucking your perineum and sacrum in with your anus soft (*Mulabandha*).

4   **Exhaling**, press your foundation, your feet, hands and shoulders down into the floor, while maintaining *Uddiyana and Mulabandha*.

5   **Inhaling**, and maintaining an active foundation, *Uddiyana* and *Mulabandha*, raise your buttocks and spine slowly off the floor.

6   **Exhaling**, lift up on to the balls of your feet.

7   **Inhaling**, bend your arms and bring your hands under your back to support your spine.

8   **Exhaling**, lower your heels to the floor.

Hold while taking each of your vertebrae away from the floor and deep into your body from your sacrum to your top spine, till ready to release to the posture indicated below according to the Series you are practising.

To maintain dynamic continuity this pose can also be entered by dropping the legs over from *Ardhasarvangasana* – first one, then the other. **64** **62**

No. 62 Ekapadasetubhujasana

One Leg Shoulder Bridge

This pose is a backbend and can therefore trouble the lumbar spine (lower back) if not approached with care. The key is correct use of the feet, keeping the back muscles soft, using the *bandhas* and activating the full length of the spine. It tones the front of the body, lengthens the front thighs and opens the chest. It teaches the importance of the elevated leg in supporting the weight of the pelvis against gravity, and is therefore a preparation for *Sarvangasana* and *Sirsasana*.

208

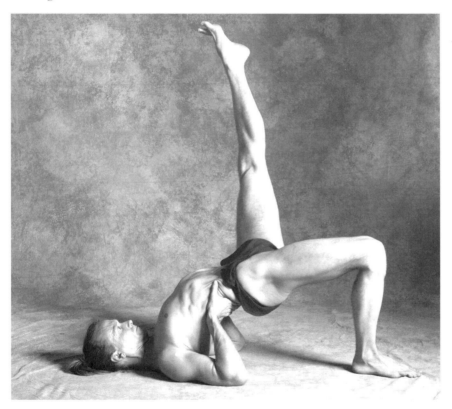

SUMMARY
Lying on your back, tuck your feet in and, keeping the shoulders and head down, raise the pelvis and arch the back, bringing the palms under for support as you lift your spine as deeply in towards the front of your body as you can. Raise one leg, keeping it straight. Keep the feet strong and maintain the *bandhas*, with your ribcrest broad, chest broad and full, with smooth, rhythmic *Ujjayi* breathing, core of the body soft.

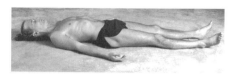

1 Lie in *Savasana*.

2 **Exhaling**, draw your heels in towards your buttocks, keeping your feet parallel, heels in line with your buttock bones.

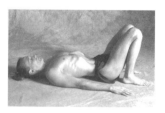

3 **Inhaling**, broaden your ribcrest and suck your solar plexus in and up so your chest becomes active, broad and full, your abdomen passive, long and empty (*Uddiyanabandha*), and flatten your pubic abdomen, sucking your perineum and sacrum in with your anus soft (*Mulabandha*).

4 **Exhaling**, press your foundation, your feet, hands and shoulders down into the floor, while maintaining *Uddiyana* and *Mulabandha*.

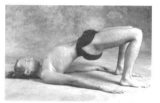

5 **Inhaling**, and maintaining an active foundation, *Uddiyana* and *Mulabandha*, raise your buttocks and spine slowly off the floor in time with your **inhalation**.

209

6 **Exhaling**, lift up on to the balls of your feet.

7 **Inhaling**, bend your arms and bring your hands under your back to support your spine.

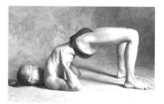

8 **Exhaling**, lower your heels to the floor.

9 **Inhaling**, lift your left knee up.

10 **Exhaling**, straighten your left leg vertically towards the ceiling, thighs sucking in, foot alive.

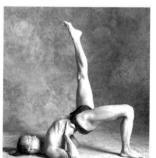

Hold while taking each of your vertebrae away from the floor and deep into your body from the sacrum to your top spine. Use your feet and legs both to keep your pelvis lifting and even. Release on an **exhalation** into *Setubhujasana*.

To maintain dynamic continuity this pose can also be entered by dropping over from *Ardhasarvangasana*.
It can also be exited to *Urdhvadhanurasana* (**63**) step 4 via *Setubhujasana* (**61**).

No. 63 Urdhvadhanurasana

Upwards Bow Pose

This pose is a strong but safe backbend. The key is correct use of the feet, keeping the back muscles soft, using the *bandhas* and activating the full length of the spine. It tones the front of the body, lengthens the front thighs, opens the chest and shoulders and develops the feet, hands and arms.

210

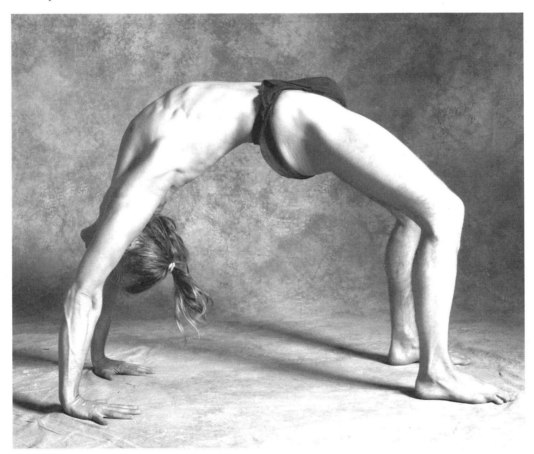

SUMMARY

From your back, with feet tucked in, hands tucked palms-down under the shoulders, straighten the arms and raise the trunk up, arching the spine deeply and fully. Keep the feet and hands strong, stable and even, maintain the *bandhas* with the chest broad and full with smooth, rhythmic *Ujjayi* breathing, core of the body soft. **64**

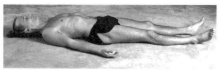

1 Lie in *Savasana*.

2 **Exhaling**, draw your heels in towards your buttocks, keeping your feet parallel, heels in line with your buttock bones.

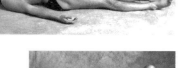

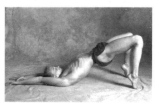

3 **Inhaling**, extend your arms alongside your ears and, raising your heels, come on to your toes.

4 **Exhaling**, bend your arms and place your palms flat on the floor underneath your shoulders, fingers pointing to your feet. Engage your palms fully, broadening the base of your fingers and the heel of your hand.

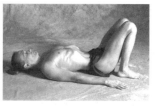

5 **Inhaling**, broaden your ribcrest and suck your solar plexus in and up so your chest becomes active, broad and full, your abdomen passive, long and empty (*Uddiyanabandha*), and flatten your pubic abdomen, sucking your perineum and sacrum in, with your anus soft (*Mulabandha*).

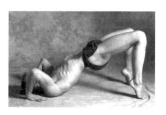

6 **Exhaling**, press your feet and hands into the floor, keeping the weight even between hands and feet, and across the surface of each of these four corners of your foundation.

7 **Inhaling**, push with your hands so that your upper body lifts and you can place the crown of your head on the floor.

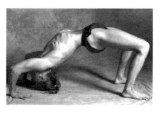

8 **Exhaling**, pressing firmly and evenly with hands and feet, and keeping your lower back soft, lift your shoulders and head off the floor, and let your head hang freely as you straighten your arms.

Hold with your foundation even and stable, while taking each of your vertebrae deep into your body from your sacrum to your top spine. Use both your feet and legs to keep your pelvis lifting and even. Release on an exhalation and roll into *Ardhapindasana*.

This pose can also be entered from *Setubhujasana* after dropping one leg from *Ekapadasetubhujasana* (**62**).

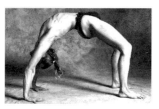

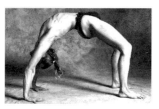

64

211

No. 64 Ardhapindasana

Half Foetus

This pose lengthens the neck and upper back muscles, rests the trunk and limb and relieves the lower back. Preparation for *Sarvangasana* and cycle. Counter-pose for backbends. It allows deep relaxation in the whole body, and soothes and refreshes the nervous system. It may be used as an opportunity to clarify *Mulabandha* (see page 50, technical section exploring Mulabandha).

212

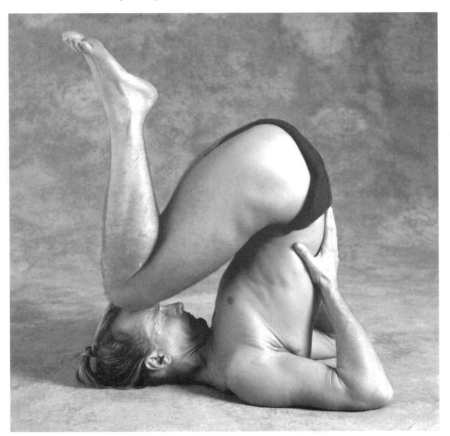

SUMMARY

From your back roll up onto your shoulders, bringing your heels into your buttocks and your palms on to your back. Maintain *Mulabandha* with the pelvic floor passive and soft as it draws in. Hold until your breath is very soft and slow, and there is no tension, hardness or holding on anywhere in your body. ✦11 ✦65 ✦67 ✦70 65 65

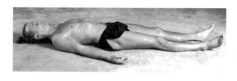

1 Lie in *Savasana*.

2 **Exhaling**, bringing your knees in towards your chest, roll back and up onto your shoulders, bringing your knees onto your forehead.

3 **Inhaling**, stretch your arms away from you behind your back, taking your shoulders away from your ears and making your neck long.

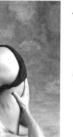

4 **Exhaling**, bring your palms on to your back and push the weight of your body further back, keeping your heels close in to your buttocks.

5 **Inhaling**, engage your pubic abdomen and suck your perineum in, keeping your anus soft (*Mulabandha*).

Hold until your breath is very soft and slow, and there is no tension, hardness or holding on anywhere in your body. Maintain *Mulabandha* with your pelvic floor passive and soft as it draws in. Release into the next posture indicated below.

213

✦ 11 ✦ 65 ✦ 67 ✦ 70 65 65

No. 65 Ardhasarvangasana

Half Shoulderstand

This is a gentle backbend that refreshes and rejuvenates the whole body. It lengthens the waist, stretches the neck and opens the chest. It teaches the correct action of the *bandhas*, which can easily be clarified in it, and how to keep the legs straight. Preparation for *Sarvangasana*. If you have neck problems, take care that this pose is actually helping you, not worsening your problem.

214

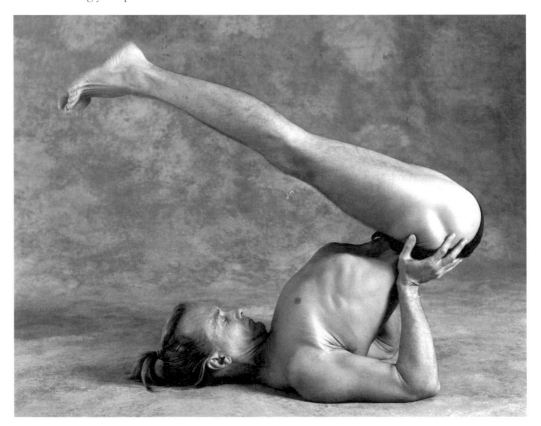

SUMMARY

From your back roll up onto your shoulders, and rolling your pelvis away with your hands supporting your back or pelvis, gently arch your back and straighten your legs. Clarify and deepen the *bandhas*, chest broad and full, ribcrest broad, abdomen long, hollow and empty, with the core of the body soft, and smooth, rhythmic *Ujjayi* breathing. ✴ 61 68 61 66

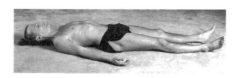

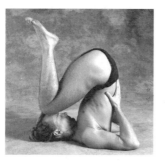

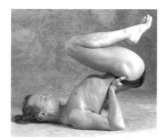

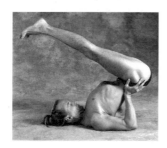

1 Lie in *Savasana*.

2 **Exhaling**, bringing your knees in towards your chest, roll back and up onto your shoulders, bringing your knees onto your forehead.

3 **Inhaling**, stretch your arms away from you behind your back, taking your shoulders away from your ears and making your neck long.

4 **Exhaling**, bring your palms on to your back and push the weight of your body further back, keeping your heels close in to your buttocks.

5 **Inhaling**, roll your knees away from you and use your hands to support your back or pelvis as you arch your back gently while lengthening your waist by taking your pelvis away from you.

6 **Exhaling**, straighten your legs so they are half way between vertical and horizontal.

215

7 **Inhaling**, broaden your ribcrest and suck your solar plexus in and up so your chest becomes active, broad and full, your abdomen passive, long and empty (*Uddiyanabandha*), and flatten your pubic abdomen, sucking your perineum in with your anus soft (*Mulabandha*).

Hold until ready to release to *Savasana*, clarifying and deepening the *bandhas* with the core of your body soft, and smooth, rhythmic *Ujjayi* breathing. Release into the next posture indicated below. 64 61 68 61 66

No. 66 Sarvangasana

Shoulderstand

This is a simple but challenging pose that rejuvenates the whole body. Alongside the Headstand it is the most nourishing pose for the body, benefiting all the internal organs, glands and nerves. It counters the lifelong effects of gravity, thereby rejuvenating every cell in the body from the shoulders to the feet. It strengthens the back muscles and the deeper muscles of the torso. It develops the arms, wrists and hands, and relieves the neck and the heart. Weight must be kept off the neck itself, and the vertebrae, by taking it on the arms and shoulder girdle. If you have neck problems, take care that this pose is actually helping you, not worsening your problem.

SUMMARY

216

From the foundation of your shoulders and elbows, and using your hands against your back, and the muscles of your trunk, elevate the whole body vertically against the pull of gravity. Keep the legs straight and strong, with no weight on the top spine or tension in the neck. Maintain the *bandhas* with the abdomen long, hollow and empty, the chest broad and full, core of the body soft with smooth, rhythmic *Ujjayi* breathing. **68**

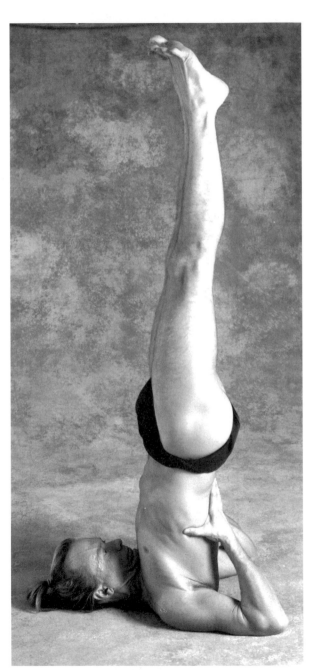

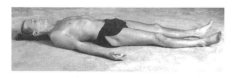

1 Lie in *Savasana*.

2 **Exhaling**, bringing your knees in towards your chest, roll back and up onto your shoulders, bringing your knees onto your forehead.

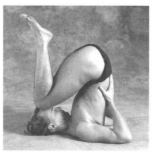

3 **Inhaling**, stretch your arms away from you behind your back, taking your shoulders away from your ears and making your neck long.

4 **Exhaling**, bring your palms on to your back and push the weight of your body further back, keeping your heels close in to your buttocks.

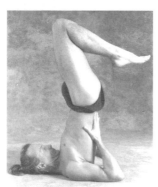

5 **Inhaling**, roll your weight away from your head, onto your hands, then lift your knees as far up and away from you as you can, keeping your legs bent.

6 **Exhaling**, lift your feet towards the ceiling, and sucking your thigh muscles in, straighten your legs and use your hands to press your spine in and up so that the whole of your body lifts up and away from your head and shoulders, bringing more weight onto your hands and your elbows. Keep your elbows as close together as you can.

217

7 **Inhaling**, broaden your ribcrest and suck your solar plexus in and up so your chest becomes active, broad and full, your abdomen passive, long and empty (*Uddiyanabandha*), and flatten your pubic abdomen, sucking your perineum in with your anus soft (*Mulabandha*).

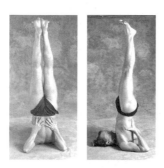

Hold with no weight bearing down on your top spine or tension in your neck. Keep the weight on hands and elbows while elevating each part of your body upwards against the pull of gravity. Release into *Halasana* (**68**). **68**

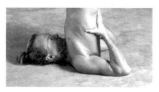

No. 67 Ardhahalasana

Half Plough

This is a soothing pose that lengthens the upper back muscles, rests the legs and heart, stretches the neck, and quietens the mind. If you have neck problems, take care that this pose is actually helping you, not worsening your problem.

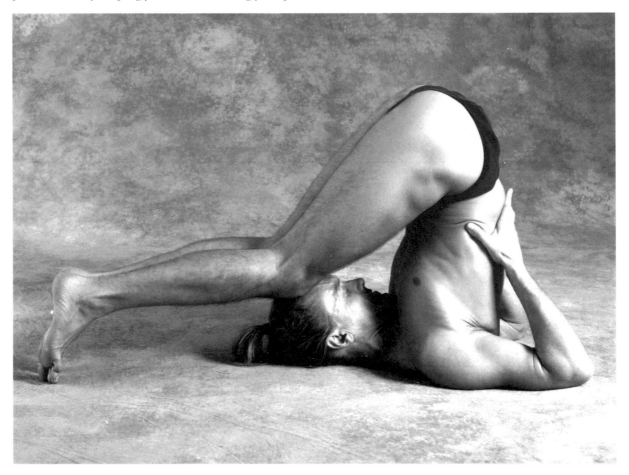

SUMMARY
From your back, roll up onto your shoulders, bringing your knees to your forehead. Bring the tips of your toes to the floor behind your head. Maintain *Mulabandha* with the pelvic floor passive and soft as it draws in. Hold until your breath is very soft and slow, and there is no tension, hardness or holding on anywhere in your body. ✦69✦

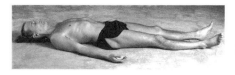

1 Lie in *Savasana*.

2 **Exhaling**, bringing your knees in towards your chest, roll back and up onto your shoulders, bringing your knees onto your forehead.

3 **Inhaling**, stretch your arms away from you behind your back, taking your shoulders away from your ears and making your neck long.

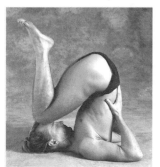

4 **Exhaling**, bring your palms on to your back and push the weight of your body further back, keeping your heels close in to your buttocks.

5 **Inhaling**, drop your feet to the floor behind your head, keeping your knees on your forehead. Make contact with the floor through the tips, not the pads or nails of your toes.

6 **Exhaling**, take your shoulders away from your ears and lengthen your neck.

219

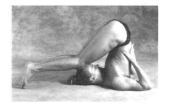

7 **Inhaling**, engage your pubic abdomen and suck your perineum in, keeping your anus soft (*Mulabandha*).

Hold with *Mulabandha* until your breath is very soft and slow, and there is no tension, hardness or holding on anywhere in your body, then release into *Karnapidasana* (**69**).

No. 68 Halasana

The Plough Pose

This is a soothing pose that lengthens the upper back muscles, tones the legs, rests the heart, stretches the neck and quietens the mind. If you have neck problems, take care that this pose is actually helping you, not worsening your problem.

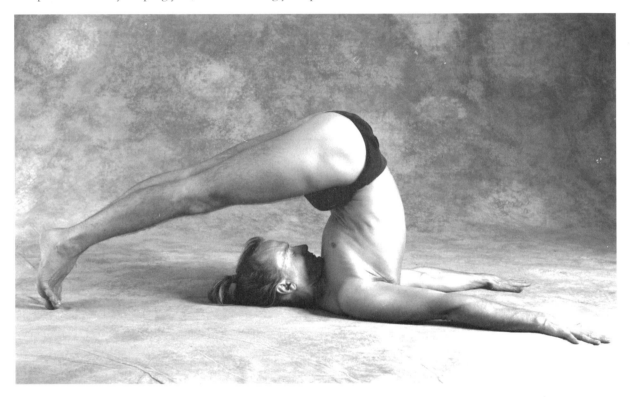

SUMMARY

From your back, roll up onto your shoulders, bringing your knees to your forehead. Bring the tips of your toes to the floor behind your head and straighten your legs. Maintain *Mulabandha* with the pelvic floor passive and soft as it draws in. Hold until your breath is very soft and slow and there is no tension, hardness or holding on anywhere in your body.

 69 69

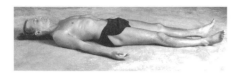

1 Lie in *Savasana*.

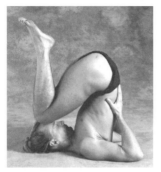

2 **Exhaling**, bringing your knees in towards your chest, roll back and up onto your shoulders, bringing your knees onto your forehead.

3 **Inhaling**, stretch your arms away from you behind your back, taking your shoulders away from your ears and making your neck long.

4 **Exhaling**, bring your palms on to your back and push the weight of your body further back, keeping your heels close in to your buttocks.

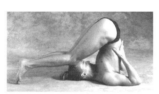

5 **Inhaling**, drop your feet to the floor behind your head, keeping your knees on your forehead. Make contact with the floor through the tips, not the pads or nails of your toes.

6 **Exhaling**, straighten your legs, sucking your thigh muscles in so that the backs of your knees open and the fronts of your legs lift away from the floor.

221

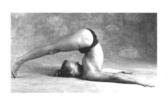

7 **Inhaling**, flatten your pubic abdomen, sucking your perineum in with your anus soft (*Mulabandha*).

8 **Exhaling**, take your arms away from your body and press your palms into the floor.

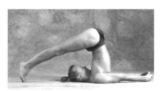

You can vary the arms position by clasping your fingers and stretching your wrists or by bringing them in the same direction as your legs and pressing the backs of your hands into the floor.

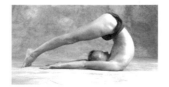

Hold with legs straight and strong, maintaining *Mulabandha*, core of your body soft, with smooth, rhythmic *Ujjayi* breathing, until ready to then release into *Karnapidasana* (**69**). 69 69

No. 69 Karnapidasana

The Foetus Pose

This pose promotes profound internalization, lengthens the back and neck muscles, rests the trunk and limbs and relieves the lower back. Counter-pose for backbends. If you have neck problems, take care that this pose is actually helping you, not worsening your problem.

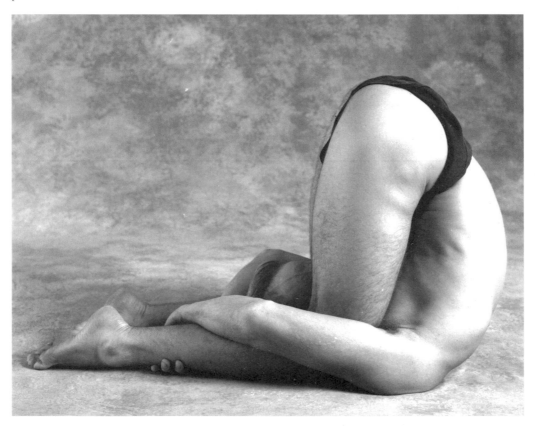

SUMMARY

From your back, roll up onto your shoulders, your arms extending alongside your ears, bringing your knees onto the forehead, then the arms, then, bending the arms, onto the wrists, and finally onto the floor by the ears while clasping the opposite shins. Maintain *Mulabandha* with the pelvic floor passive and soft as it draws in. Hold until your breath is very soft and slow, and there is no tension, hardness or holding on anywhere in your body.

  70 70

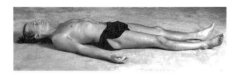

1 Lie in *Savasana*.

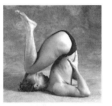

2 **Exhaling**, bringing your knees in towards your chest roll back and up onto your shoulders, bringing your knees onto your forehead.

3 **Inhaling**, stretch your arms away from you behind your back, taking your shoulders away from your ears and making your neck long.

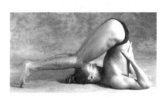

4 **Exhaling**, bring your palms on to your back and push the weight of your body further back, keeping your heels close in to your buttocks.

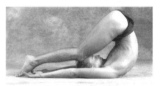

5 **Inhaling**, drop your feet to the floor behind your head with your knees on your forehead and extend your arms alongside your ears. Hold for a while with smooth, rhythmic *Ujjayi* breathing.

223

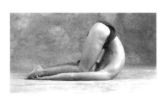

6 **Exhaling**, drop your knees onto your upper arms, and let your feet rest on your hands, keeping your whole body relaxed. Hold for a while with smooth, rhythmic *Ujjayi* breathing.

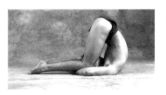

7 **Exhaling**, bend your arms and bring your hands together, then draw your knees onto your wrists and interlace your fingers just past your head, and let your feet rest on your hands, keeping your whole body relaxed.

Hold for a while with smooth, rhythmic *Ujjayi* breathing.

8 **Exhaling**, drop your knees onto the floor by your ears and, bringing your arms over your calves, cross your wrists as you lightly grip the opposite shins, keeping your whole body relaxed.

Hold until your breath is very soft and slow, and there is no tension, hardness or holding on anywhere in your body, then release into the posture indicated below. ✦64 70 70

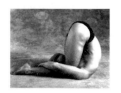

No. 70 Ardhamatsyasana

Half Fish

This pose lengthens the throat and waist, opens the chest and gently arches the back. If you have neck problems, take care that this pose is actually helping you, not worsening your problem. It is a counter-pose to the Shoulderstand cycle. The more you lift the top spine, the more the neck will let go.

224

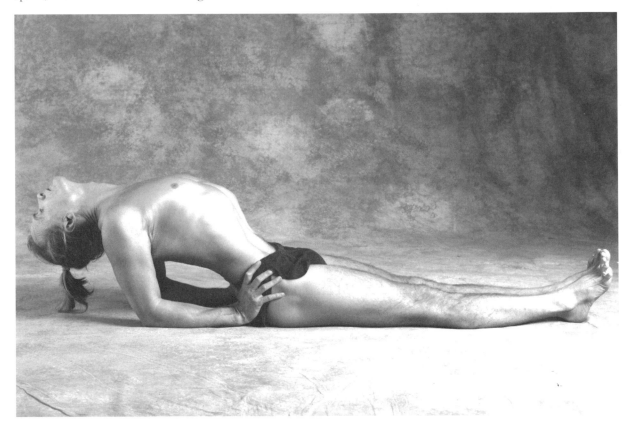

SUMMARY

Sitting with legs in front, straight and strong, lean back onto your elbows, fingers on your hipbones, taking your head back and lifting and opening your chest. Maintain the *bandhas*, chest broad and full, abdomen long hollow and empty, core of the body soft, with smooth, rhythmic *Ujjayi* breathing. **73** one of **73** **75** **76** **77** or **78** **72**

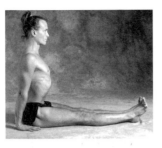

1 Sit on the floor with legs outstretched, straight and strong, feet together and alive, with your spine lifting straight out of your pelvis (*Dandasana*).

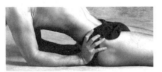

2 **Inhaling**, lean back and bring your elbows, one at a time, to the floor behind you, and put your hands on your hips so your thumbs are behind your fingers coming round the side of your hipbones to the front.

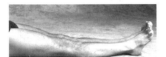

3 **Exhaling**, make your legs straight and strong, your feet alive.

4 **Inhaling**, pressing your elbows down, lift and broaden your ribcrest, sucking your solar plexus in and up so that your chest is broad and full, your abdomen long, hollow and empty (*Uddiyanabandha*), and flatten the pubic abdomen, with your anus soft as you suck your perineum and sacrum in (*Mulabandha*).

225

5 **Exhaling**, lift your chin up slightly and press the base of your skull forwards and up, and

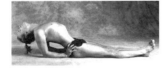

6 **Inhaling**, as you gently arch your back, take your head back and down in as wide an arc as possible, keeping as much space as possible in the back of your vertebrae.

Hold, keeping your abdomen long, empty and hollow, your chest high, broad and full with your legs strong and feet alive. When ready, release to the posture indicated below.

73 one of 73 75 **76** 77 or 78 72

No. 71 Balasana

Child Pose

This pose pacifies the whole body, especially giving relief to the lower back. Preparation for dog pose. Counter-pose to backbends and Headstand. The buttocks are not in between the heels in this pose, but resting on them. It teaches the spirallic action of the arms necessary to *Adhomukhasvanasana*.

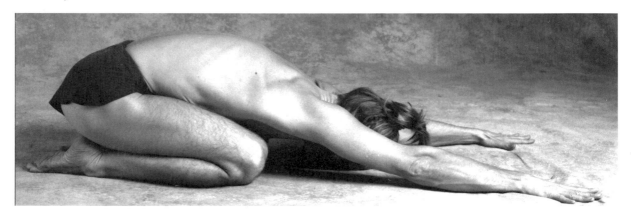

226

1 From all fours, slip your toes back so that the tops of your feet come to the floor and drop your buttocks back down onto your heels, your chest down on to your knees.
2 Keeping your buttocks down on your heels, extend your arms forwards till they are straight and shoulder-width apart.
3 Broaden your palms and lengthen your fingers as you press your palms into the floor shoulder-width apart.
4 Lengthen your arms out of your shoulders, keeping the shoulderblades broad and, as you press the ball of your thumbs down, spiral your upper arms to create space between your shoulders and your neck.
5 Flatten your pubic abdomen, sucking your perineum in, with your anus soft (*Mulabandha*).

Hold till ready to release, continually lengthening and straightening your arms. To make the pose more passive, extend your arms back, palms up alongside your feet, and then relax completely. Come up when ready to enter the next posture.

SUMMARY
Sit on the heels and bring the chest down onto the knees, extending the arms alongside the ears, pressing with the palms to straighten the arms. Suck your perineum in with your anus soft.

One of **76** **77** or **78**

Balasana may also be entered from *Adhomukhas-vanasana* ((**15**), page 114) by bending the legs to bring the shins to the floor while slipping the toes back so that the tops of the feet come to the floor, and dropping the buttocks back down onto the heels, the chest down onto the knees.

No. 72 Sirsasana

Headstand

This is a simple but challenging pose, that must be done with a rigorous precision to protect the neck. This is mostly with regard to establishing and maintaining the foundation of the pose: head, hands, elbows and forearms. It powerfully rejuvenates the whole body, benefiting all the internal organs, glands and nerves. Alongside the Shoulderstand it is the most nourishing pose for the body. It reverses the lifelong effects of gravity, replenishing every cell in the body. It strengthens the deeper muscles of the torso, the respiratory muscles and the lungs. It develops the arms, wrists and hands, realigns the neck, and relieves the heart. Weight must be kept mostly on the arms and elbows. If you have neck problems, take care that this pose is actually helping you, not worsening your problem. Each part of the body, except the foundation, must be activated against gravity to lift its own weight. No specific instructions are given for using the breath. Use what you have learned of breath/body synchronization from the other postures. Breathe freely into the pose so that your breathing supports you. Do not hold or force your breath.

SUMMARY

With your head cradled by your hands and your weight supported by the crown of your head, forearms and wrists, extend the whole body vertically against the pull of gravity so that you make a straight vertical line with shoulders lifting as you press the foundation firmly down. With a strong charge in the legs and feet, maintain the *bandhas*, chest broad and full, abdomen long, hollow and empty, core of the body soft with smooth, rhythmic *Ujjayi* breathing. **71**

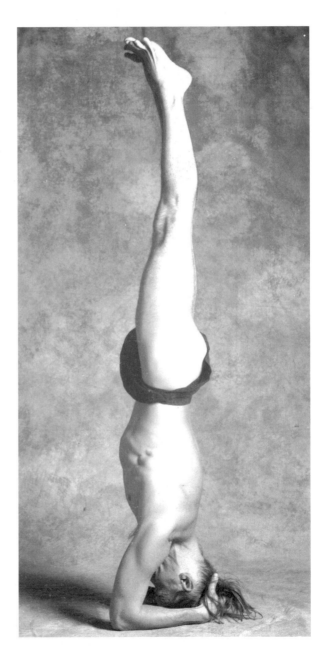

227

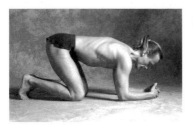

1   Sitting on your heels, knees bent, feet under your buttocks, locate the crown of your head by finding a small indentation where the lines between the ears and from the bridge of the nose cross just in front of the ridge that runs across the top of the head.

2   Interlacing the fingers deeply but loosely, make the thigh bones parallel to each other so that your inner thighs slightly separate, and place your elbows on the floor so that the inner edges of your elbows embrace the outer knees. (If your knees are in line with each other, your elbows will be in line. It is important that one elbow is not even 1 millimetre in front of the other. This occurs if you wrap your fingers round your elbows to put them on the floor the right distance apart. This leads to a slight but significant twisting of the neck which eventually creates muscular imbalance and tension in the neck. If your knees are in line, with the thigh bones parallel, and the inner elbows are wrapping the outer knees, the elbows will be the correct distance apart.)

228

3   Press the outer edge of your wrists firmly into the floor, keeping the forearm bone vertical and pressing down, so that the ball of the thumbs do not roll out and down towards the floor.

4   Place the crown of your head on the floor within the space created by your hands, making a gentle hemispherical curve, so that the balls of your thumbs and your top fingers are gently embracing the back of your head. The lower, smaller fingers will not be in contact with your head. The balls of your thumbs will be against the skull near its base at your ears. Pressing in firmly with the balls of your thumbs, keep your fingers relaxed, and press down with the outer edge of the wrists and forearm bones so that your forearm bones remain vertical.

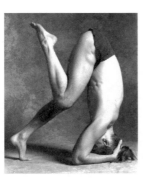

5   Straighten your legs so your buttocks rise, and walk your feet gently in towards your head so that your back lifts towards a vertical line. Be careful not to walk in so far that the weight rolls off the crown towards the back of your head. Keep your shoulders lifting away from your ears by pressing the outer edge of the wrists and forearm bones firmly into the floor while pressing the balls of the thumbs firmly into your skull.

6   Slowly raise one foot off the floor and draw its knee tight into your chest, keeping your heel tight into your buttock.

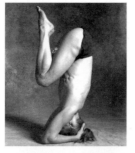

7 Raise the second knee tight into your chest alongside the first and bring its heel tight into your buttock.

8 Keeping your knees and feet together and your legs bent, raise your knees as high as you can towards a vertical line, so your shins and feet hang behind your thighs. Press the outer edge of your wrists and forearm bones firmly into the floor while pressing the balls of your thumbs firmly into your skull; keep weight on the elbows.

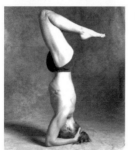

9 Lift your feet, keeping them together till your legs are straight and vertical, lifting your shoulders away from your ears as you press the outer edge of your wrists and forearm bones firmly into the floor while pressing the balls of your thumbs firmly into your skull, keeping weight on your elbows.

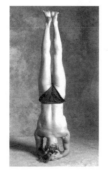

10 **Inhaling**, broaden your ribcrest, sucking your solar plexus in and up so that your chest is broad and full, your abdomen hollow, long and empty (*Uddiyanabandha*), and flatten your pubic abdomen, sucking your perineum in with your anus soft (*Mulabandha*). Keep your shoulders soft and lifting away from the floor.

229

Maintain the *bandhas* with a strong charge in the legs and feet, core of the body soft with smooth, rhythmic *Ujjayi* breathing. Release by bending your legs, knees into your chest, and taking first one foot to the floor, then the other, then coming to child pose. **71**

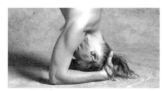

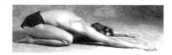

No. 73 Sukhasana

Easy Pose

This pose is the simplest of sitting poses, and can be used for meditation when the joints in the lower body are restricted. Be sure you allow no pressure or pain in the knees, nor dropping into the lumbar spine. It opens the joints of the legs.

230

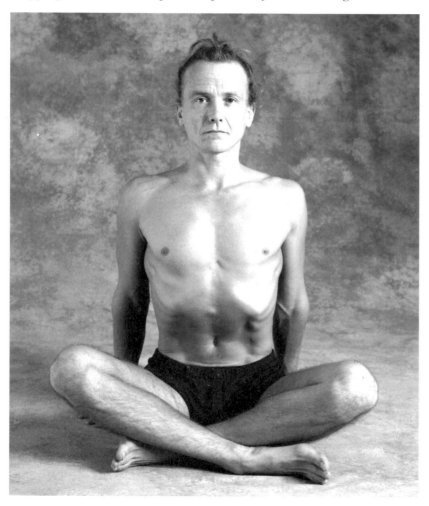

SUMMARY
Sit with legs crossed, each foot supporting the opposite leg. Relax the trunk, lengthen the spine and sit quite still.

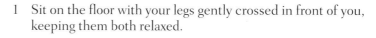

1 Sit on the floor with your legs gently crossed in front of you, keeping them both relaxed.

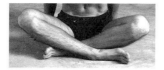

2 Adjust the position of your feet so that each foot rests under and supports the opposite leg. One will be in front, one behind.

3 Relax your legs, your pelvic floor, your abdomen, your shoulders and your face.

4 Place your palms flat behind your buttocks and make sure that your hip bones are just slightly forwards of your buttock bones so that your lower back is not rounded. Keep the weight even on the foundation provided by your shin and buttock bones.

5 Lift your chest and lengthen your spine, taking your breastbone away from your pelvis, your armpits away from your hips. Relax your shoulders.

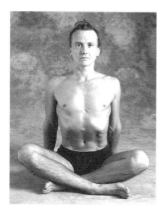

6 Lengthen your neck and gaze ahead and slightly down. Keep your face relaxed, eyes and ears soft. Soften the core of your body completely.

231

Remain motionless until ready to release into *Savasana*.

Please refer to the instructions entitled GENERAL INSTRUCTIONS FOR SITTING AT THE END OF YOUR PRACTICE (page 242).

Every other day, cross your legs the other way round, so that the joints develop equally on left and right.

No. 74 Urdhvasukhasana

Upwards Pose

This pose is an extension of *Sukhasana*, and supports the inhalation in an easily attained position. When tired it can be held instead of an active *vinyasa* in between poses. It opens the chest and mobilizes the neck. Counter-pose to forward extensions.

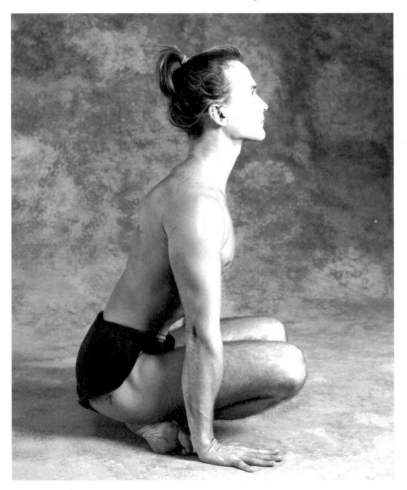

SUMMARY
Sit with legs crossed, each foot supporting the opposite leg, and bring your arms around your shins, palms to the floor. Then roll your weight off your buttocks and onto your palms and feet. Look forwards with smooth, rhythmic *Ujjayi* breathing.

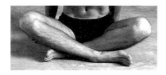

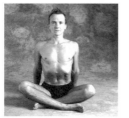

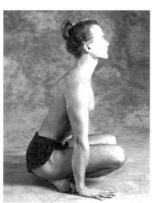

1   Sit on the floor with your legs in front of you, keeping them both relaxed.

2   Adjust the position of your feet so that each foot rests under and supports the opposite leg. One will be in front, one behind.

3   Relax your legs, your pelvic floor, your abdomen, your shoulders and your face.

4   Bring your arms round the outside of your thighs and place your palms on the floor.

5   Rolling your weight forwards on to your palms and feet and off your buttocks, lift your chest and lengthen your spine. Relax your shoulders.

6   Look straight ahead and lengthen your spine more and open your chest fully.

7   Soften the core of your body completely.

Remain motionless until ready to release into *Dandasana* (**32**).

Every other day, cross your legs the other way round, so that the joints develop equally on left and right.

233

No. 75 Virasana

Hero Pose

This is a powerful sitting pose that opens the backs of the knees and ankles, strengthens the arches of the feet and stabilizes the sacrum. It can damage the knee ligaments if done clumsily or before you are ready. If your buttocks cannot reach the floor, support them on your heels or the balls of the big toes, until they can.

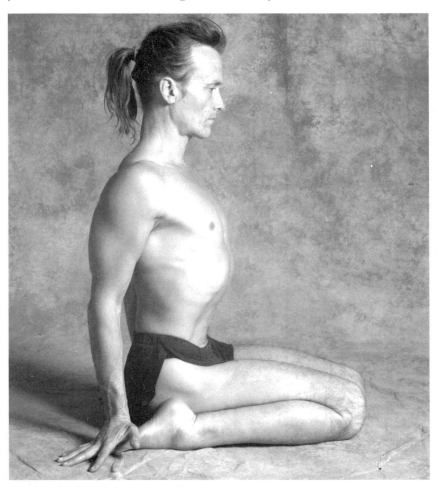

SUMMARY
Sit with buttocks in between the feet. Relax the trunk, lengthen the spine and sit quite still.

1

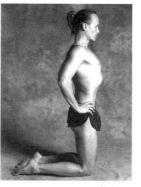

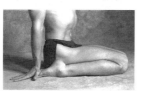

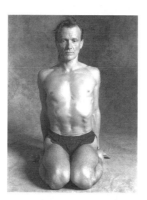

1 Sit kneeling on the floor.
2 Raise your buttocks till your thighs are perpendicular.
3 Separate your feet and knees till they are as wide as your buttock bones, with the tops of your feet spread on the floor, your inner and outer ankle bones both the same height from the floor.
4 Lengthen your inner ankle, bringing the inner edge of your foot into the line of the inner edge of your shinbone so that the toes of your feet are not curving in towards each other. Keep the length from your inner shinbone to your inner heel.
5 Lower your buttocks till they rest on the floor in between your feet.
6 Use your fingers to separate your toes so that they are all individually pressing into the floor.
7 Keep your thigh bones parallel to each other and tuck the outer edges of your shinbones in and under so your inner knees lift, without lifting your buttocks.
8 Press the heels of your hands onto the outer edges of your feet to maintain the alignment of your shinbones and knees.
9 Lift your chest and lengthen your spine, taking your breastbone away from your pelvis, your armpits away from your hips. Relax your shoulders.
10 Lengthen your neck and gaze ahead and slightly down. Keep your face relaxed, eyes and ears soft. Soften the core of your body completely.

Remain motionless until ready to release your legs into *Savasana*.

1

Please refer to the instructions entitled GENERAL INSTRUCTIONS FOR SITTING AT THE END OF YOUR PRACTICE (page 242).

IF YOUR BUTTOCKS DON'T REACH THE FLOOR, USE YOUR FEET OR YOUR HEELS TO SUPPORT THEM. DO NOT TURN THE FEET OUT IN THE WAY THAT CHILDREN DO WHILE SITTING LIKE THIS.

235

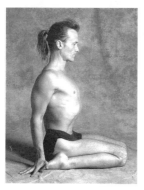

No. 76 Ardhasiddhasana

Half Adepts Pose

This is a simple, stable sitting pose attainable by most people. It develops the back muscles, opens the hips, loosens the ankles, centres energy and stabilizes the mind. Preparation for *Padmasana*.

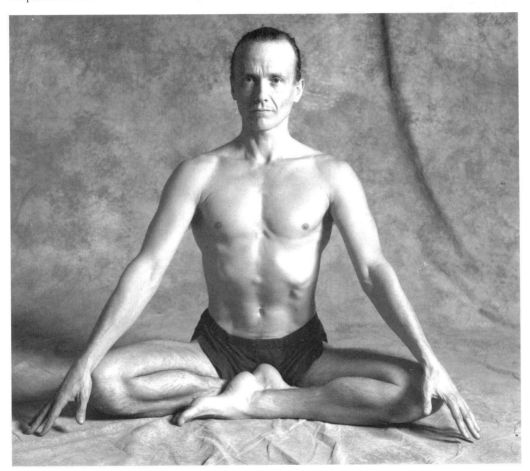

SUMMARY
Sit with legs crossed, one heel in front of the other in line with the centre of the pubic bone. Relax the trunk, lengthen the spine and sit quite still. 🔳 ⬤

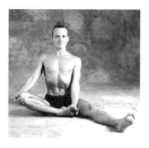

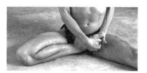

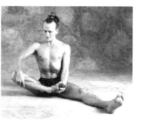

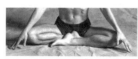

1 Sit on the floor with your legs in front of you, keeping them both relaxed.
2 Take hold of your right leg by the knee and the heel, keeping it relaxed.
3 Supporting the weight of your leg in your left hand on the heel, use your right hand to pull the flesh of the calf and thigh up towards you so that the bones of your thigh and shin can come closer together.
4 Use both hands to bring your shin bone as tightly in against your thigh bone as possible, making sure that you do not twist your shinbone up towards your face.
5 Put your right heel on the floor in front of the centre of your pubic bone. Relax your ankle and your knee.
6 Bend your left leg in the same way and put your left heel just in front of your right so that your feet are touching.
7 Relax your legs, your pelvic floor, your abdomen, your shoulders and your face.
8 Make sure that your hip bones are just slightly forwards of your buttock bones so that your lower back is not rounded. Keep the weight even on the foundation provided by your shin and buttock bones.
9 Lift your chest and lengthen your spine, taking your breastbone away from your pelvis, your armpits away from your hips. Relax your shoulders and place your hands on your knees.
10 Lengthen your neck and gaze ahead and slightly down. Keep your face relaxed, eye and ears soft. Soften the core of your body completely.

237

Remain motionless until ready to release into *Savasana*.

Please refer to the instructions entitled GENERAL INSTRUCTIONS FOR SITTING AT THE END OF YOUR PRACTICE (page 242).

Every other day, cross your legs the other way round, so that the joints develop equally on left and right.

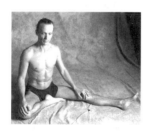

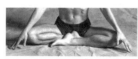

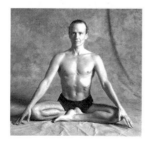

1　**1**

No. 77 Siddhasana

Adepts Pose

In its classical form, with the lower heel pressing your perineum, the upper heel the genitals, this is the most potent *asana* alongside *Padmasana* for energetic transformation, *Pranayama*, meditation and psychological transmutation. It develops the back muscles, open the hips and chest, loosens the ankles, centres energy and stabilizes the mind. Preparation for *Padmasana*.

238

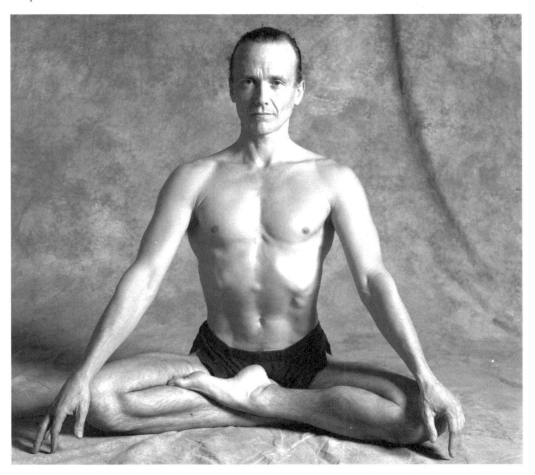

SUMMARY
Sit with legs crossed, one heel on top of the other in line with the centre of the pubic bone. Relax the trunk, lengthen the spine and sit quite still.

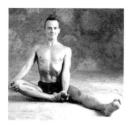

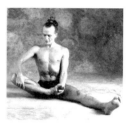

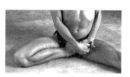

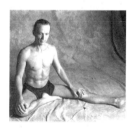

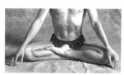

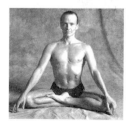

1 Sit on the floor with your legs in front of you, keeping them both relaxed.
2 Take hold of your right leg by the knee and the heel, keeping it relaxed.
3 Supporting the weight of the leg in the left hand on your heel, use your right hand to pull the flesh of the calf and thigh up towards you so that the bones of your thigh and shin can come closer together.
4 Use both hands to bring your shin bone as tightly in against your thigh bone as possible, making sure that you do not twist your shinbone up towards your face.
5 Put your right heel on the floor in front of the centre of your pubic bone. Relax your ankle and your knee.
6 Bend your left leg in the same way and put your left heel on top of your right heel.
7 Relax your legs, your pelvic floor, your abdomen, your shoulders and your face.
8 Make sure that your hip bones are just slightly forwards of your buttock bones so that your lower back is not rounded. Keep the weight even on the foundation provided by your shin and buttock bones.
9 Lift your chest and lengthen your spine, taking your breastbone away from your pelvis, your armpits away from your hips. Relax your shoulders and place your hands on your knees.
10 Lengthen your neck and gaze ahead and slightly down. Keep your face relaxed, eyes and ears soft. Soften the core of your body completely.

Remain motionless until ready to release into *Savasana*.

Please refer to the instructions entitled GENERAL INSTRUCTIONS FOR SITTING AT THE END OF YOUR PRACTICE (page 242).

Every other day, cross your legs the other way round, so that the joints develop equally on left and right.

239

No. 78 Padmasana

Full Lotus

The quintessential yoga posture. It is the most potent *asana* alongside *Siddhasana* for energetic transformation, *Pranayama* meditation and psychological transmutation. It develops the back muscles, opens the hips and chest, loosens the ankles, centres energy and stabilizes the mind. Care must be taken that the ligaments of the top knee are not strained by trying to force it down. You can place a cushion, blanket or book under it until flexibility in your hips allows it to rest naturally on the floor. Great care must be taken in placing and removing the top knee so that no damage is done to the ligaments.

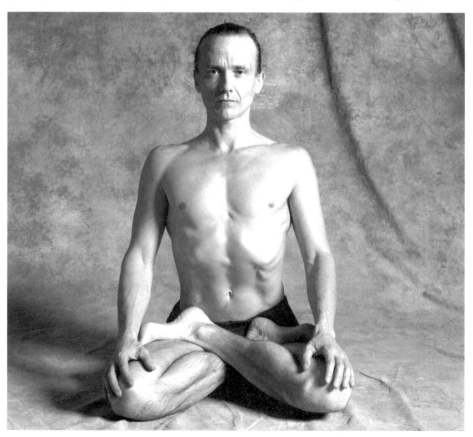

SUMMARY
Sit with legs crossed, each foot at the root of the opposite thigh. Relax the trunk, lengthen the spine and sit quite still. **1** **1**

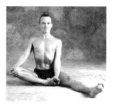

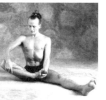

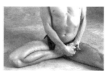

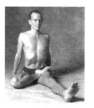

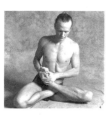

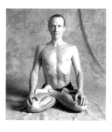

1 Sit on the floor with your legs in front of you, keeping them both relaxed.

2 Take hold of your right leg by the knee and the heel, keeping it relaxed.

3 Supporting the weight of the leg in the left hand on the heel, use your right hand to pull the flesh of the calf and thigh up towards you so that the bones of your thigh and shin can come closer together.

4 Use both hands to bring your shin bone as tightly in against your thigh bone as possible, making sure that you do not twist your shinbone up towards your face.

5 Move your right thigh bone close to the left, and as your right foot draws near to your left thigh, place it at the top of your thigh with the heel near the navel.

6 Bend your left leg in exactly the same way, using both hands to support, and releasing the flesh from between calf and thigh.

7 Bring your left thigh towards your right so your left foot moves towards your right hip, carefully taking your left foot over your right leg until your left foot rests at the root of your right thigh.

8 Gently pull your thighs closer together, bringing your heels more tightly into your navel.

9 Make sure that your hip bones are just slightly forwards of your buttock bones so that your lower back is not rounded.

10 Lift your chest and lengthen your spine, taking your breastbone away from your pelvis, your armpits away from your hips. Relax your shoulders and place your hands on your knees.

11 Lengthen your neck and gaze ahead and slightly down. Keep your face relaxed, eyes and ears soft. Soften the core of your body completely.

Remain motionless until ready to release into *Savasana*.

Please refer to the instructions entitled GENERAL INSTRUCTIONS FOR SITTING AT THE END OF YOUR PRACTICE (page 242).

Every other day, cross your legs the other way round, so that the joints develop equally on left and right. 1 1

General Instructions for Sitting at the End of Your Practice

At the end of your practice, after the inversions, you will come to a sitting posture. It is here that the effects of your practice are fertilized. The fertilizer you use is conscious breathing. Spend as much time as you can sitting still and breathing consciously. Allow this to occur in the following *Vinyasa Karma*. Try it now. Go slowly through the steps. Build up from 2 minutes per step to 10. If some are longer, some shorter, so be it. Don't force it, if it's working for you, you will want to spend more time with it

Step 1
Sitting still, with spine elevated without strain by the *bandhas*, allow your whole body to relax. Release *Uddiyana* and *Mulabandha*. Do not drop your chest or slump your spine. Focus on releasing your throat and jaw, your pelvic floor and your abdomen especially. As you focus on your abdomen feel it relaxing deeply. As it relaxes, feel the movement of your abdominal wall increasing gradually and freely with each inhalation and exhalation. Stay a while.

Step 2
Gradually focus your attention more and more closely and deeply onto the floating ribs. Feel them opening and expanding outwards as you inhale, falling in again as you exhale. Do not force your breathing. Allow it to flow freely. Ignore the abdomen, letting it be as it is. As you make deeper and deeper contact with the floating ribs, encourage them, openly and without force, to very slowly and very gradually open a little more with each inhalation. Do not force this. You are simply inviting whatever dormant capacity you have to awaken in its own time. It will do so, but especially in the beginning it will do so more if allowed to do so slowly. The respiratory muscles are not only

chronically underused, but loaded with emotional tension. Respect this temporary state. You are about to change it. Do so gently. Once you have clearly reached your current capacity, maintain your breathing until the rhythm becomes absolutely fluid and effortless. This will be characterized by a slow, fine breath flowing consistently without strain, jerkiness or changes in speed. Allow this effortless rhythm to enhance your awareness with its integrity. If you feel resistance, feel the resistance, but continue if you can. If you feel release, feel the release, but continue.

Step 3

Shift your focus away from the floating ribs to the top chest. Ignore the floating ribs, letting them be as they are. As you make deeper and deeper contact with the fixed ribs, encourage them, openly and without force, to very slowly and very gradually open a little more with each inhalation. Do not force this. You are simply inviting whatever dormant capacity you have to awaken in its own time. It will do so, but especially in the beginning it will do so more if allowed to do so slowly. The respiratory muscles are not only chronically underused, but loaded with emotional tension. Respect this temporary state. You are about to change it. Do so gently. Once you have clearly reached your current capacity, maintain your breathing until the rhythm becomes absolutely fluid and effortless. This will be characterized by a slow, fine breath flowing consistently without strain, jerkiness or changes in speed. Allow this effortless rhythm to enhance your awareness with its integrity. If you feel resistance, feel the resistance, but continue if you can. If you feel release, feel the release, but continue. If your chin wants to go down to the breastbone, allow it to do so without dropping your chest.

Step 4

Allow your awareness to embrace the abdomen, floating ribs and fixed ribs. As you make deeper and deeper contact with the lungs, encourage them, openly and without force, to very slowly and very gradually open a little more with each inhalation. Do not force this. You are simply inviting whatever dormant capacity you have to awaken in its own time. It will do so, but especially in the beginning it will do so more if allowed to do so slowly. The respiratory muscles are not only chronically underused, but loaded with emotional tension. Respect this temporary state. You are about to change it. Do so gently. Once you have clearly reached your current capacity, maintain your breathing until the rhythm becomes absolutely fluid and effortless. This will be characterized by a slow, fine breath flowing consistently without strain, jerkiness or changes in speed. Allow this effortless rhythm to enhance your awareness with its integrity. If you feel resistance, feel the resistance, but continue if you can. If you feel release, feel the release, but continue.

Step 5

Gradually and slowly reverse the *Vinyasa* steps **4, 3, 2, 1** until you are breathing normally again. Stay a while.

Step 6

Slowly lift your chin. Clarify and stabilize your posture effortlessly. Relax deeply without collapsing the spine or chest. Focus on releasing your throat and jaw, your pelvic floor and your abdomen especially. Allow your awareness to embrace the flow of sensations that results from the fact of your breathing. Make no attempt to influence your breathing in any way at all. Let it be. Stay a while simply following the changing sensations of your breathing. If any sensations or feelings arise persistently and overwhelmingly, allow your awareness to embrace and penetrate them fully, using the flow of your breathing to maintain your focus.

Step 7

Clarify and stabilize your posture effortlessly. Relax deeply without collapsing the spine or chest. Focus on releasing your throat and jaw, your pelvic floor and your abdomen especially. Allow your awareness to embrace the flow of sensations that results from the fact of your having a body. Feel the changing play of sensation as you sit there. Make no attempt to influence this in any way at all. Let it be. Feel whatever you feel just as and when you feel it. Do not deliberately add anything. If you need to, use the flow of your breathing to maintain your awareness in a stable, clear focus on what is actually occurring. If any sensations or feelings arise persistently and overwhelmingly, allow your awareness to embrace and penetrate them fully, using the flow of your breathing to maintain your focus. Stay a while.

Step 8

Clarify and stabilize your posture effortlessly. Relax deeply without collapsing the spine or chest. Allow your awareness to embrace the flow of your perception, sensations, feelings, thoughts, images, that result from the fact of your having a mind. Attend the changing play of perception as you sit there. Make no attempt to influence this in any way at all. Let it be. Perceive whatever you perceive just as it is. Do not deliberately add, change, hold or resist anything. If you need to, use the flow of your breathing to maintain your awareness in a stable, clear focus on what is actually occurring. If any perceptions arise persistently and overwhelmingly, allow your awareness to embrace and penetrate them fully, using the flow of your breathing to maintain your focus. Stay a while. After a while, just sit there doing absolutely nothing at all. Allow the mind to absorb all perceptions freely, without preference or imposition. It does not matter if the mind is full of thoughts. Just let it be. Let yourself be. Experience yourself just as you are. Enjoy yourself just as you are. Eventually come out of your sitting posture and lie in *Savasana* (*1*).

IV

The Practice of Dynamic Yoga

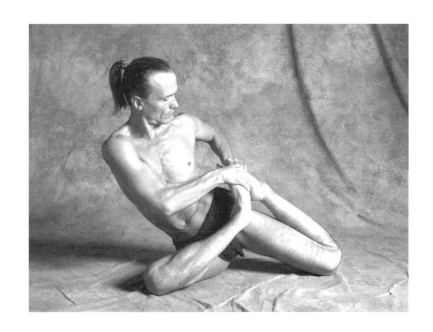

13

THE PACIFYING SERIES ✸

The Pacifying Series is designed to clarify the fundamentals of the Hatha Yoga method. It does so within the context of very simple postures, accessible to all. No matter how experienced you are please start with the Pacifying Series.

The Foundation Series introduces the basic standing postures, and develops the dynamic of the Hatha Yoga method within the context of the simple postures. It should be practised until all of the postures come without effort.

The Preparatory Series presents most of the postures of the traditional Yoga Chikitsa sequence. The more extreme ones are omitted. It is more demanding in terms of flexibility and stamina than any other Series. Even when you are comfortable practising the Preparatory Series, there will be times, when you are tired or stressed, when it will be too much for you. Then practice one of the other two Series, or one of the less advanced shorter sequences.

The six shorter sequences are for when you have less time available than required for the longer Series.

246

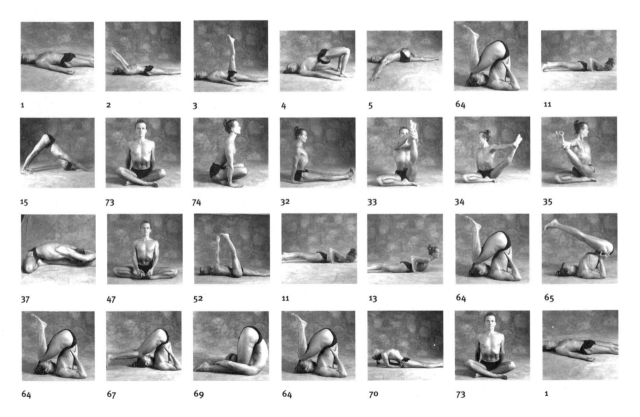

THE FOUNDATION SERIES ■

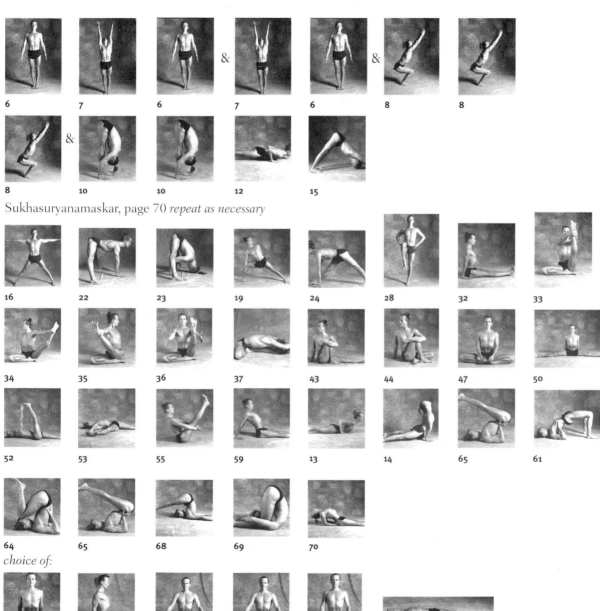

Sukhasuryanamaskar, page 70 *repeat as necessary*

choice of:

THE PREPARATORY SERIES ●

Suryanamaskar, page 72 *repeat as necessary*

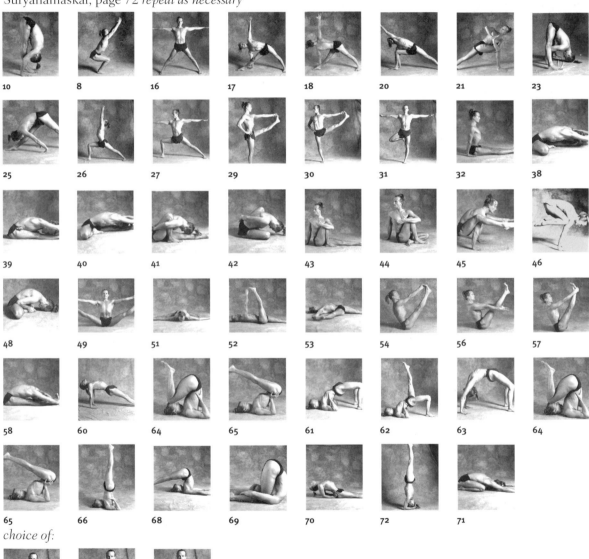

10   8   16   17   18   20   21   23

25   26   27   29   30   31   32   38

39   40   41   42   43   44   45   46

48   49   51   52   53   54   56   57

58   60   64   65   61   62   63   64

65   66   68   69   70   72   71

choice of:

76   77   78

THE SHORT PRACTICES

Please note: *vinyasa – your choice as to which kind.*

Dynamic Practice 1

Suryanamaskar, page 72
repeat as necessary

10
8
20
21
25
26
27
29
30
32
vinyasa
54
56
57
56
59
60
vinyasa
64
65
61
62
63
64
69

Dynamic Practice 2

Suryanamaskar, page 72
repeat as necessary

10
8
32
vinyasa
54
56
57
56
59
60
vinyasa
64
69

Dynamic Practice 3
(Advanced Students Only)

6 & 7
6 & 8
9 & 10
23
19
24
28
32
13
vinyasa
14
vinyasa
65
61
63
64
72
71
1

Passive Practice 1

1
2
3
4
5
15
64
65
64
67
69
64
70
73
1

Passive Practice 3
(Advanced Students Only)

15
10
8
72
71
15
65
66
68
69
66
70
78
1

Passive Practice 2

15
10
8
64
65
64
67
69
64
70
73
1

GLOSSARY

adhara	support
adho	downwards, down
ardha	half
Asana	yoga posture, the practice of yoga postures
asana	the inner activity of the body in yoga postures, process of adjusting the body to awaken cellular intelligence
ashtanga	eight limbs
Ashtanga Yoga	the yoga of the eight limbs, referred to by Patanjali in the Yoga Sutras
Ashtanga Vinyasa Yoga	a Hatha Yoga system derived from the Yoga Korunta by T. Krishnamacharya and K. Pattabhi Jois of Mysore
aswini	mare's mouth
Aswini mudra	mare's gesture
baddha	bound
baka	crow
bala	child
Bandha	seal, grip, lock or energetic relay
bhakti	devotion, ecstatic love, adoration
Bhakti yoga	the yoga of worship
bhuja	shoulder
chakra	vibrational frequency, resonating in body areas
chatura	four
chikitsa	therapy, remedial process
Desikachar T. K.	contemporary Yoga Master, son of Krishnamacharya
drushti	point of concentration
Drushti	directed attention
dwi	two
eka	one
Gherandasamhita	a mediaeval Hatha Yoga text
ha	solar current, active energy, creative principle
hala	plough
hasta	arm, hand
hatha	balancing of opposites energies, intense energizing
Hatha Yoga	the yoga of energetic balancing
Hathayogapradipika	a mediaeval Hatha Yoga text
Iyengar B. K. S.	contemporary Yoga Master, brother-in-law of Krishnamacharya

Iyengar Yoga	Hatha Yoga system based on the postures in the Yoga Korunta, devised and taught by B. K. S. Iyengar. The most well-known style of Hatha Yoga.
Jala	net
Jalandhara Bandha	net supporting lock of the throat, separating cranium from trunk
jnana	wisdom, insight
Jnana Yoga	the yoga of inner enquiry
karma	action, action and reaction
Karma Yoga	the yoga of service
karna	ear
kona	angle
krama	step
Krishnamacharya T.	modern Yoga Master with incomparable impact on yoga in the west through his senior students, and his championing of the Yoga Korunta and its unique emphasis on Vinyasa.
kurma	tortoise
Marichya	a historical yoga master, or sage
Matsyendra	a mediaeval Hatha Yoga master
mudra	gesture, seal or energetic circuit
mukha	face
mula	root, base
Mulabandha	root lock, base seal, root relay
Muladhara	root chakra, base energetic resonance centre
nava	boat
pada	leg, foot
parsva	side, flank
parivrtta	twisting
pascima	west-facing aspect, rear, back of the body
Patanjali	an ancient codifier of yoga, author of Yoga Sutras
Pattabhi Jois K.	contemporary Yoga Master, Krishnamacharya's senior student whom he instructed to master and transmit the Yoga Korunta teachings
pida	pressure
Power Yoga	Hatha Yoga system popular in America derived from Ashtanga Vinyasa Yoga
prana	life force, vital energy, breath
Pranayama	the practice of energetic regulation through the breath
pranayama	refining the breath
purva	east-facing aspect, or front of the body

raja	royal
Raja Yoga	the yoga of meditation
sadhana	spiritual practice
samadhi	a state of consciousness in which subject, action and object are united in revelation of their true nature
sarva	all of, the whole
sarvanga	the whole body
setu	bridge
shakti	pure and applied energy, manifest divinity, the active energy of consciousness
sirsa	head
siva	pure consciousness, transcendent divinity, source of manifest energy
Sivasamhita	a mediaeval Hatha Yoga text
soma	sweet, immortalizing nectar dripping from deep inside the skull tasted and channelled in the throat
sukha	easy
sutra	thread, aphorism, verse
tan	stretch, lengthen
tha	lunar current, passive energy, receptive principle
tri	three
trikona	triangle
Ud	upwards
Uddiyana Bandha	rising energy seal, upwards flying grip
Ujjayi	victorious, powerful
Ullola	wave
urdhva	upwards
ut	intense
uttana	intense stretch
utthita	extended
Vajroli mudra	an esoteric energy practice involving the orgasm carrying nerve
vinyasa	progression, continuity
Vinyasa	a continuity sequence of breath-linked poses
vinyasa krama	step-by-step progression
Vinniyoga	Hatha Yoga system devised by Krishnamacharya on the principle of Vinyasa Krama derived from the Yoga Korunta. Now taught by his son Desikachar and his students.
Virabhadra	the name of a mythical warrior
yama	regulate, refine, extend, adjust, restrain

yana	flying
yoga	the state of union, the process of realizing union
Yoga Korunta	an ancient yoga manual, used by Krishnamacharya, source of Ashtanga Vinyasa Yoga method
Yoga Sutras	an ancient yoga manual compiled by Patanjali
yogasana	yoga posture

Asana Glossary
(A word-for-word translation)

ADHOMUKHASVANASANA	downwards facing dog pose
ARDHACHATURANGADANDASANA	half-four limbs staff pose
ARDHAHALASANA	half-plough pose
ARDHAMATSYASANA	half-fish pose
ARDHAPADMASANA	half-lotus pose
ARDHAPARSVATTONASANA	half-intense side stretch pose
ARDHAPINDASANA	half-embryo pose
ARDHAPURVOTTANASANA	half-intense front stretch pose
ARDHASARVANGASANA	half-whole body pose
ARDHASIDDHASANA	half-power pose
ARDHURDHVAMUKHASVANASANA	half-upward facing dog pose
ARDHUTTANASANA	half-intense stretch pose
BADDHAKONASANA	bound angle pose
BAKASANA	crow pose
BALASANA	child pose
BHUJADHANURASANA	shoulder bow pose
CHATURANGADANDASANA	four limbs staff pose
DANDASANA	staff pose
DWIHASTABHUJASANA	two arms shoulder pose
EKAPADANAVASANA	one leg boat pose
EKAPADANGUSTASANA	one big toe pose
EKAPADAPASCIMOTTANASANA	one leg intense back stretch pose
EKAPADASANA	one leg pose
EKAPADASETUBHUJASANA	one leg shoulder bow pose
EKAPADASUPTAPARIVRRIASANA	one leg supine twist pose
HALASANA	plough pose
JANUSIRSASANA	knee head pose
KARNAPIDASANA	ear pressure pose
MARICHYASANA	sage's pose
MERUDANDASANA	holy mountain staff pose

NAMASKARPARVRITAPARSVAKONASANA	greeting revolved side angle pose
NAVASANA	boat pose
PADMAPASCIMOTTANASANA	lotus back intense stretch pose
PADMASANA	lotus pose
PADOTTANASANA	leg intense stretch pose
PARSVAIKAPADANGUSTASANA	side one big toe pose
PARSVAIKAPADASANA	side one leg pose
PARSVAKONASANA	side angle pose
PARSVAVIRABHADRASANA	side warrior's pose
PARSVOTTANASANA	side intense stretch pose
PARIVRRIAIKAPADASANA	twisting one leg pose
PARIVRRIAMARICHYASANA	twisting sage's pose
PARIVRRIASUKHAMARICHYASANA	twisting easy sage's pose
PARIVRRIATRIKONASANA	revolving triangle pose
PASCIMOTTANASANA	back intense stretch pose
PURVOTTANASANA	front intense stretch pose
SALAMBAPARSVAKONASANA	supported side angle pose
SARVANGASANA	whole body pose
SAVASANA	corpse pose
SETUBHUJASANA	shoulder bow pose
SIDDHASANA	power pose
SIRSASANA	head pose
SUKHAMARICHYASANA	easy sage's pose
SUKHAPADAPASCIMOTTANASANA	easy leg back intense stretch pose
SUKHANAVASANA	easy boat pose
SUKHASANA	easy pose
SUKHASURYANAMASKAR	easy sun salutation
SUKHAVINYASA	easy continuity sequence
SUKHULLOLA	easy wave
SUPTAHASTASANA	supine arm pose
SUPTAPADASANA	supine leg pose
SUPTAPARSVAPADANGUSTASANA	supine side big toe pose
SUPTURDHVAPADANGUSTASANA	supine raised big toe pose
SURYANAMASKAR	sun salutation
TADASANA	mountain pose
TRIKONASANA	triangle pose
UBBAYAPADAHASTASANA	both foot hand pose
UBBAYAPADANGUSTASANA	both big toe pose
UPAVISTAKONASANA	seated angle pose
URDHVABADDHAKONASANA	upwards bound angle pose
URDHVADHANURASANA	upwards bow pose
URDHVAIKAPADASANA	upwards one leg pose

255

URDHVAKONASANA	upwards angle pose
URDHVAMUKHASVANASANA	upward facing dog pose
URDHVAPADOTTANASANA	upwards intense leg stretch pose
URDHVASUKHASANA	upwards easy pose
URDHVAHASTASANA	upwards arms pose
UTKTASANA	fierce pose
UTTANASANA	intense stretch pose
UTTHITATRIKONASANA	extended triangle pose
VINYASA	continuity sequence
VIRABHADRASANA	warrior's pose
VIRASANA	hero pose
VRIKSASANA	tree pose

ABOUT THE AUTHOR

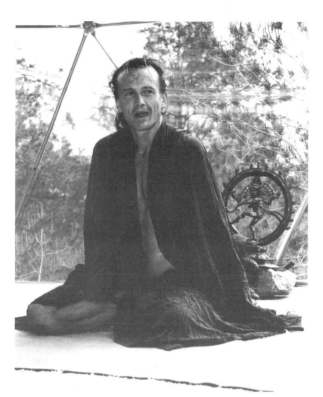

Godfrey began his practise of Hatha Yoga in 1973, having observed his uncle, an Anglican minister, praying in Vriksasana. Although he has studied widely, with many teachers of many styles, he has always found his most important guidance on his mat or his cushion. He began teaching in 1979, and has taught full time since 1989. He currently runs a residential yoga training centre on the island of Ibiza, Spain, where he lives. Since 1990 he has been studying with Roshi Soten Genpo, leader of the largest Zen Sangha in the West. He, more than anyone else, has helped Godfrey to clarify the true nature of self, reality and yoga.

If you would like to

- know about dynamic yoga teacher training
- organize a dynamic yoga workshop or retreat
- purchase dynamic yoga audio tapes, video tapes and practise charts

or if you wish to be kept informed of Godfrey's teaching schedule via an annual mailout, please write to Godfrey at:

36 Stanbridge Road
London SW15 1DX
or
Can Am des Puig
Sant Mateu 07816
Ibiza Spain
or
email info@windfireyoga.com
(Your name and address will be kept on computer unless you inform us that you prefer otherwise.)

For more information about Godfrey's activities, please visit our website at www.windfireyoga.com.